THE
30-DAY WAY
TO A
BORN-AGAIN
BODY

THE
30-DAY WAY
Joy Gross
TO A
BORN-AGAIN
BODY

A Total Regimen Plus the

New Natural Carbohydrate Diet

That Can Make You

Stay Thinner,

Look Younger, Live Longer

RAWSON, WADE PUBLISHERS, INC. NEW YORK

BLACK-AND-WHITE PHOTOGRAPHS by Brian Hamill

Library of Congress Cataloging in Publication Data
Gross, Joy.
The 30-day way to the born again body.
Includes index.
1. Reducing diets.   2. Health.   I. Title.
RM222.2.G74   613.2'5   78-54690
ISBN 0-89256-067-3

Published simultaneously in Canada by McClelland and Stewart, Ltd.
Manufactured in the United States of America
by American Book–Stratford Press
Saddle Brook, New Jersey

Designed by Helen Barrow
Third Printing February 1979

*To the memory of my mother, Genevieve,
whose beauty, intelligence and nonconformity
were my initial inspiration.*

ACKNOWLEDGMENTS

I am *most* grateful to Colette Dowling, without whose expertise, talent, co-ordination, dedication, hard work, and encouragement this book could not have happened; to Robert Gross, from whom I've learned so much, who helped me with the physiological material in the book and who lent his support in many other ways; to my cousin Yvonne Adrian for her contribution to the exercise chapter; to my children, Debbie, Wendy, Louis, David, and Betsy for their patience and understanding and to my son-in-law Brian Hamill not only for the cover photo, but for his encouragement as well; to Lowell Miller for *his* encouragement; to Gabrielle Dowling for the typing she did; to Alpha-Graphics in Hyde Park, N.Y., for the charts and graphs; and to all the wonderful guests from Pawling Manor who led me to the realization of the need for this book—my warmest thanks to all of you.

CONTENTS

SECTION I: THE BORN-AGAIN BODY

1.	*Why I Wrote This Book*	3
2.	*Food for a New Body: The Story of How I Changed My Life*	7
3.	*What You Will Learn from This Book*	12
4.	*Secrets for Living Longer . . . and Better*	16
5.	*The Dynamic New Natural Carbohydrate Diet*	22
6.	*A New Solution for the Overweight*	36
7.	*Fasting to Look Younger (and Lose Weight)*	44

SECTION II: YOUR NEW LIFETIME EATING PLAN

8.	*Your New Lifetime Eating Plan*	59
9.	*Drinking and Health*	72
10.	*How to Make Your New Diet a Way of Life*	80
11.	*How to Pick Perfect Fruits and Vegetables*	85
12.	*Ten Salads You Can Eat All You Want of and Still Lose Weight*	95
13.	*Dynamic Natural Carbohydrate Recipes*	101
14.	*A Month of Born-Again Menus with Calorie and Protein Count*	119

SECTION III: BORN-AGAIN LIVING

15. *Exercise: Shape Up and Live Longer*   141
16. *The Breath of Life*   159
17. *Sun: The Super Energizer*   167
18. *Four Kinds of Rest for Health and Beauty*   171
19. *Your Body Responds to Happiness*   177
20. *Born-Again Desire*   183

SECTION IV: YOUR 30-DAY BORN-AGAIN BODY
PROGRAM

21. *30 Days to a New You*   193

SECTION V: THE QUESTIONS I'M ASKED MOST
FREQUENTLY

22. *Frequently Asked Questions*   235

APPENDICES
*Appendix A: Recommended Fasting Retreats, Vacation Retreats, and
    West Coast Consultants*   241
Appendix B: Mail Order Sources for Fruits, Vegetables, and Nuts 242
Appendix C: Protein Counter   243

INDEX   255

THE
BORN-AGAIN
BODY

CHAPTER 1

Why I Wrote This Book

Like so many others, perhaps you've arrived at that day of reckoning when you look in the mirror and find yourself admitting, "Things aren't working out the way I want them to. My youthfulness and energy are slipping between my fingers. I don't *feel* as well as I should. I don't *look* the way I'd like. I wish I could start over again."

Well, you can.

THIS BOOK IS FOR PEOPLE OF ANY AGE WHO FEEL THEY'RE LIVING (AND LOOKING) BELOW PAR AND WOULD LIKE A FRESH START. If you've ever said to yourself in even the smallest, innermost whisper, "I wish I could have another chance," this book can help. I call it "The Born-Again Body" precisely because my own and the experience of many others has proved that when you change your diet and institute healthful new practices in your life, you will end up looking and feeling brand-new.

Change is a funny thing. You have to *want* it, first. And before you can want it, you have to admit that life isn't completely satisfying for you the way it is, that things are not what they might be. Because we're proud, such an admission isn't always easy to make. In fact, it takes *courage*. But it's the first big step, the step without which nothing else can happen. Once you've said the magic words, "I want more!" it's like unleashing a log jam. All sorts of possibilities that once were tied up and inaccessible will become available to you. Anything can happen!

IT'S POSSIBLE TO START OVER. It's possible to abandon those negative living patterns—the things you do (or don't do) that have been weighing you down and contributing to your energylessness, those vague aches and pains, the loss of that fresh, vibrant smile that used to greet you whenever you looked in the mirror. The loss of your supple, slender body.

IT'S POSSIBLE TO STRIKE THOSE LIFE-DENYING HABITS RIGHT OFF THE BOOKS. I know, because I've done it. I can help you. As you read through the pages of this book, you will learn how to drop negative patterns and substitute new, positive ones that will bring you the ultimate reward, all around good health. You will improve your appearance, your physical strength, your level of energy to such a degree that you will both look and feel like a different person.

It isn't as difficult as you might imagine. I have brought about remarkable changes in my life and have witnessed remarkable changes in the lives of many others. For two decades now, I've worked with my husband, Robert Gross, at Pawling Health Manor, which we run in Hyde Park, New York. I have seen people turn their lives from unhealthy, low-energy states of sterile existence into robust, exciting, pleasure-packed adventures. I have seen the people who are continually drained by chronic, low-grade illnesses become free of sickness, beautiful and whole. These people often say they feel as if they've been born all over again. They achieve their miraculous new lives by changing their diets and by following a new, total regimen.

YOU CAN REVOLUTIONIZE YOUR ENTIRE APPROACH TO LIVING. The information I have to give you is based on knowledge and firsthand experience. If I have learned one thing during my years of helping people to improve their health and appearance at the Manor, it's that crash diets and "quickie" solutions don't work. To "go on a diet" is a false idea, a fragmented, superficial approach to health and beauty. It's like staying up all night to cram for an exam. You may pass the test, but what you learned won't stay with you for very long.

Scientists have really got interested, of late, in finding new ways to increase our health and longevity. They've discovered—and subsequently studied—little known cultures where people live far longer than we do and remain youthfully robust and productive, dying not from devastating diseases, but gently, naturally, simply because the total organism has gradually worn down. We have much to gain by applying this new information to our lives. It's possible to change everything—the way you look, the way you feel, the energy you have, your resistance to illness and fatigue. It all goes together, and it all affects the ultimate concern, which is the number of years you have for living your life.

THERE'S NO MIRACULOUS PILL OR VITAMIN, NO MAGICAL "DRINK," BUT THERE IS A WAY! It's nature's way—the kind of diet and total health regimen we were meant by nature to follow. Interestingly, it's the kind of regimen that people in some technologically less developed areas follow—while living happily and healthily into their hundreds.

True health is wholeness. It's having everything—mind, body, and spirit—in a beautiful state of balance. To get to that state, to be "born again," you must first learn how to nourish your body the way nature intended it to be nourished. In a word, that means learning how to eat all over again.

Next, and of almost equal importance, is relearning the use of your body. The kind of society we live in has made us sedentary. You must learn ways of flexing, exercising, and toning your body until it becomes the marvelously strong, energetic organism it was designed to be. This involves knowing proper breathing techniques as well, so you can be sure to get the full supply of oxygen your body needs. (You'd be surprised by the number of people who drag along, breathing incorrectly and getting far less oxygen than the body really needs.)

Before starting off on your new diet and Born-Again Body Program you should have a complete rest and detoxification program. At Pawling Health Manor we help people to do this through fasting. It's possible, however, to fast for short periods at home.

That's one of the reasons I decided to write this book. People look and feel so terrific when they leave Pawling Health Manor that thousands have come to me and asked for something they can follow at home, so that they can *continue* looking and feeling terrific.

For these people, and for *anyone* who wants to lose weight, feel better, and look just great, I have organized a fully detailed program. It's a plan for optimum health, looks, and energy. Step by step I'll show you how to get off your old, unhealthy food addictions and onto a new diet of live (natural!) carbohydrates. *Also, by learning to control your protein intake, it's actually possible for you to slow down the aging process and live longer.*

There's a lot that's new for you to learn about, but when you begin following my 30-day program everything that you discover in this book will fall into place. Almost automatically you'll find yourself on a new track, one that will provide you with more hours, days, and years to accomplish the things in life that make you happy.

CHAPTER 2

Food for a New Body: The Story of How I Changed My Life

A surprising number of people, some with quite serious health problems, have turned their lives around as a result of applying new, radically simple rules of health to their daily living. I say "new" not because these rules come out of some advanced technology (on the contrary), but because lately we've gone way off the track as far as knowing how to live the good life. Everything that relates to health has been made to seem tremendously complicated, and we are told our livelihoods depend on shoving lots of substances into our bodies—medicines, vitamins, "supplements," and so on. That's not true.

Much of what I am about to tell you is simplicity itself, but it's far different from the way most people live today. Once you've read through it, I'm sure the whole Born-Again Body Program will impress you as making amazingly good sense simply because it *is* so natural, so lacking in anything artificial or strange.

THE EXPERIENCE THAT TURNED MY LIFE AROUND, THAT RE-TURNED ME TO A SIMPLE, NATURAL STATE OF HEALTH, GAVE ME NEW ENERGY, A VIBRANT APPEARANCE, AND HAS KEPT ME FEELING YOUNG AND EXHILARATED FOR MANY YEARS, OCCURRED WHEN I WAS QUITE YOUNG. Fifteen, to be exact. I had a particular health problem that pushed me toward a way of life that seemed quite drastic, at the time, though it soon became as smooth and easy as the motion of the tides.

What I learned, the way of life I took up, can make enormous changes in anyone's life. You don't have to have a special health condition, as I did, to take a turn that will be almost miraculously for the better. I'm going to tell you my story (briefly) because it shows what *anyone* can accomplish. And because if you *do* happen to have a health-related problem, my story may give you hope.

How I Became Born Again

If you're not normally attractive and healthy at the age of fifteen the experience can be something so vivid that its memory will continue to motivate you the rest of your life. That is what happened to me.

I grew up in the small village of Hazelwood, in the mountains of North Carolina. When I was seven, my mother complained to our local doctor that I was a nervous child. When I was nine she took me to see him because I'd developed a peculiar, scabby condition on my skin. We soon found out that I had a disease for which there was no known cause and no known cure, a disease that had turned the lives of millions to misery: psoriasis. "Your daughter will just have to learn how to live with it," he said, and gave us a tube of salve that did little more than make my hair limp and stringy. For several years the psoriasis remained more or less confined to my scalp. Not until later would the embarrassing patches of skin begin to cover my entire body.

After a while a new neighbor, a widow whose name was Margaret, and her children moved in next door to us. Margaret's husband had died of a heart attack when he was quite young. Margaret had begun reading everything she could find about health and nutrition. She was worried about her children. The doctor had told Margaret her husband's early death had been abetted by the rich foods he ate.

MARGARET'S SEARCH LED HER TO THE DISCOVERY OF A SYSTEM OF HEALTH CARE THAT ADVOCATED PERIODIC FASTS AND A DIET OF NATURAL, WHOLE FOODS. My mother, with health and weight problems of her own, became fascinated. When mother saw how much Margaret's health had improved once she came back from a fasting institution and had begun preparing healthier meals for her family, she decided to give it a try herself. (That decision of hers was to change my life.)

WE COULD HARDLY BELIEVE IT WAS MOTHER WHEN SHE AR-
RIVED HOME FROM HER FAST! She fairly danced into the house,
more sparkly-eyed, smooth-skinned, and thinner than I ever re-
membered seeing her. Best of all, her energy and enthusiasm knew
no bounds.

VAST CHANGES WERE MADE IN OUR HOUSEHOLD. Mother threw
out the white sugar, white flour, and any and all products made
from either. She decided that meat, poultry, and fish would be
served only rarely. Menus became streamlined. Fresh fruits and
vegetables were the featured items. At that time she became interested in the teachings of a small but lively group of people called
Natural Hygienists, who advocate eating this way.

Children often resist change, at least initially. At school I would
always try to swap my lunch of fruit for someone else's peanut-butter-and-jelly sandwich. Whenever a nickel or dime would come my
way I'd clutch it fiercely and run to Mr. McCoy's corner store to
load up on silverbells, chocolate bars, and marshmallows. I was not
going to be cheated out of the finer things in life!

AS I GREW OLDER, MY "CHEATING" KEPT MY PSORIASIS GOING.
It wasn't until I was fourteen, however, that I really did myself in.
That summer I went to visit relatives in Lost Creek, Kentucky,
where my dad had grown up on a farm. There my aunts delighted
in stuffing me with the things I couldn't get at home—banana
pudding, ice cream, toast dripping with butter, and deep fried
chicken.

As the summer progressed, I noticed that my "bumps" were no
longer confined to my scalp, but had begun appearing along my
hairline. Soon I noticed the pesky little scabs in my eyebrows, my
ears, along the edges of my nostrils. Spots began to pop out on my
arms, legs, belly, chest, and back. I began to panic. I found excuses
not to go swimming. I tried to cover the bright red patches on my
face with make-up, but to no avail. The patches that were flat at
the beginning of the day had turned bumpy by evening.

By the time I arrived back home at the end of the summer, I
was a mess. The situation made me terribly depressed. Sometimes I
felt so sorry for myself I even thought about suicide. "I look like a
freak, a sideshow curiosity," I would think to myself. "What good is
a life like this?"

Finally, I began to do some thinking about all the things my mother had been trying to teach us for so long. I wanted desperately to be normal. No taste thrills were worth this agony.

I DECIDED TO CHANGE TO MY MOTHER'S WAY OF EATING. I went on a fast to get my system cleansed of the toxins and impurities built up by the refined sugars and other processed foods I'd been eating. Fasting helped to break the addiction I had to these destructive foods. It also prepared my body to respond optimally to the new kinds of foods I'd be putting into it.

After a week I broke the fast and began my new diet: fresh fruits and vegetables, some nuts and raw seeds, very small quantities of grain. What I was doing was lowering by half or more the amount of protein I'd been consuming; at the same time I was vastly increasing my consumption of natural (not processed) carbohydrates. This was a way of eating taken up before the turn of the century by a group of people who, like my mother (who had joined the group), called themselves Natural Hygienists. For years I followed this eating plan, defending myself against people who found it strange. But now, excitingly for everyone, established nutritional research groups have caught up with the hygienists. Recently the U.S. Senate's Select Committee on Nutrition and Human Needs has shown that Americans consume far more protein than is good for them. It has told us to cut down on protein (especially animal protein) as well as fats and sugars, and to eat more of the natural carbohydrates—fruits, fresh vegetables, seeds, and nuts.

THERE ARE CERTAIN IMMUTABLE LAWS THAT GOVERN LIFE AND HEALTH. When these laws are broken, disease and early aging result.

Just as it takes time for organs to break down and chronic disease to establish itself, so it takes time to reverse the aging process and allow regeneration to take place. It took months for my skin to clear, but clear it did—and it stayed that way! Imperceptibly, at first, the scales became thinner, the edges began to fade, the spots became smaller. At the end of nine months on my new eating regimen, all that was left of the psoriasis were a few vaguely pink areas, and in time, those, too, faded.

Anyone who's ever had psoriasis knows how tenacious it is. Just because my skin had cleared didn't mean that I could then return to an unhealthy way of eating and living. This wasn't a short-term "diet," something to adhere to for a while and then abandon. Whenever I deviated, warning spots broke out on my face. Quickly I'd go back to my fruit and vegetable regime, fast for a few days, or go on pure citrus or watermelon, or fresh juice for a day or two, to clean my system of toxins and give it a rest.

HEALTH AND LONGEVITY RESULT FROM A TOTAL WAY OF LIFE. I found out about cholesterol, and that my system couldn't handle it. (Doctors now tell us that women are only *relatively* immune to heart and blood-vessel disease and that cholesterol is something on which men and women both have to cut down.) I became a vegetarian. I also began a vigorous program of daily exercise and found ways of getting regular exposure to sunlight, even in winter, so my body could synthesize its own vitamins.

What I discovered was that the very same diet and way of life that got my psoriasis under control helps to prevent disease in general, and has kept me looking and feeling younger than others my age. As I studied and began doing work in the field of nutrition I learned the reasons for this. The metabolism of certain foods causes much more wear and tear on the body than the metabolism of other kinds of foods. This wear and tear promotes disease and early aging. The truth is, human beings can live much longer and enjoy more health, energy, and good looks than most of us do. Nor is this something that can be decided only by fate.

You can make that decision yourself and it can affect the length and quality of your life.

CHAPTER 3

What You Will Learn from This Book

"THE BORN-AGAIN BODY" PROGRAM WILL TEACH YOU A WHOLE NEW WAY OF EATING FOR THINNESS, GOOD LOOKS, AND LONGEVITY. I call it the Natural Carbohydrate Diet. Mounting government research shows we've been eating the wrong way in this country for a long time. Protein foods are not the gold we've assumed them to be, nor are carbohydrates the dross. In fact it's quite the opposite. The government is telling Americans to cut back on protein and drastically boost the amount of natural (unprocessed) carbohydrate in their diets.

IN THIS BOOK YOU WILL LEARN A BRAND-NEW FORM OF DIETARY CONTROL. Others have told you to count calories and carbohydrate grams. I am going to tell you how to count protein.

Excess protein puts on weight and its metabolic process (especially that of animal protein) actually is aging, so you *must* know how much protein you're consuming and how *not* to overconsume. I will show you how to determine exactly how much protein you *should* be eating for your weight and age, and how to cut down to that amount. You will learn to use a special Protein Counter that will show you, by grams, how much protein is contained in the foods you eat. You will learn how to tally up these grams in order to stay on the safe side with your PI (Protein Intake).

AT THE SAME TIME YOU WILL LEARN HOW TO BOOST YOUR INTAKE OF NATURAL CARBOHYDRATES AND NATURAL SUGARS. I will tell you how protein metabolism works, how carbohydrate metabolism works, and why the latter is easier on you and less aging. You will learn which foods are acid-forming and must be omitted from the diet. You will learn how to combine your foods for the least wear and tear on your internal organs. And best of all, you will learn how you can eat more, more, more of the low-density carbohydrates and not gain weight!

I WILL GIVE YOU ALL THE INFORMATION YOU NEED FOR SWITCHING TO THE DYNAMIC NEW NATURAL CARBOHYDRATE DIET. There are even special pots to use for proper steaming of your foods. Yet however radically it will change your life, your New Lifetime Eating Plan is really simplicity itself. My whole family follows this very same plan (the children have followed it since they were born!) and we are all slender, high-energy people who are virtually never sick.

My husband and I are also far younger looking than most people our age. The picture you see of me on the cover was taken just before this book was published. I am fifty years old. Most people eat in a way that causes them to look old before their time. I have absolutely no doubt that when you change the way you eat you can stay young looking longer, and even turn back the clock and look younger than you do right now. This is not so far-fetched as it might sound. You know people who have aged terrifically when under excessive stress, only to look younger again when the burden is removed from their lives. Well most people in this country *eat* in such a way as to keep themselves in a state of unnecessary stress. Change the eating, get rid of the stress, and you'll look and feel younger, I guarantee it.

THE EATING PLAN THAT HAS BEEN SO GOOD FOR ME IS DESCRIBED IN DETAIL IN THIS BOOK. You'll see that it's very different from the way you eat now. My family and I take no vitamin pills, nor do we need to. We make use of the sun and other of nature's aids to help our bodies synthesize whatever vitamins we don't get directly from our foods. We avoid all chemicals. Our ways of coping with stress are nature's ways.

The way we eat, including the fact that all of us—including my adolescent daughters—fast from time to time, has given us finely tuned "appestats."

The natural carbohydrates we eat give us a great deal of pleasure. With our natural appestats, we know when we are truly hungry, and we eat only then. Food tastes utterly delicious to us, and is thoroughly satisfying.

FASTING IS THE FIRST STEP TO LOOKING YOUNGER. Many people fast for weight loss (and you can, too) but I am even more excited by fasting's rejuvenating effects. It has an almost miraculous potential for making you look better and feel higher, healthier, more vitalized. I will tell you exactly what to do to cleanse your body of stored toxins and tune up your metabolism with a Total Water Fast. It's the most efficient way of breaking your addiction to destructive foods and preparing your body for optimal response to your new way of eating.

With certain exceptions, which I'll list later, most people can safely manage a short fast at home, as long as they learn the basic principles of the fasting metabolism first. I will give you the biophysical information you should have before going on a fast by yourself. Then I'll tell you exactly how to proceed, including what you should eat and drink a day or two before you begin your fast, and a re-feeding plan for when you end it. I'll discuss the safety and effectiveness of fasting, in general, and address specific questions such as whether or not you can exercise, go to work, travel, and drive a car while fasting.

TO HELP YOU INCORPORATE ALL THESE CHANGES INTO YOUR DAILY LIFE I'VE PUT TOGETHER A WONDERFUL, 30-DAY PLAN—THE BORN-AGAIN BODY PROGRAM. It will take you by the hand and lead you through the morning, noon, and night of every day for a month. You will go on two short fasts, one at the beginning of the month and one at the end. In between, I will show you how to begin eating in a brand-new way. Your new Natural Carbohydrate Diet will make you *feel* brand-new—lighter, less fatigued, powerfully in charge of your life. You will also get in the habit of exercising your body, day by day, to get it looking the way it was meant to look. To relax naturally and relieve stress you will learn breathing and meditating techniques. Most important of all, I will teach you *how to think positively* and consciously about everything you're doing, every step you're taking, every negative pattern in your life that you're facing . . . and conquering!

Here is a preview of how the Born-Again Body Program works:

» Each morning of the program begins with a Mindset that gives techniques for helping you change your goals and *psyche yourself into action.*

» Each day of the program lists a Food Plan telling you exactly *what to eat and drink* for that day. (Or, should it be a day that falls during one of the two short fasts, what you should do to fast and feel comfortable.)

» Each day tells you which *exercises* to do. There are also *natural grooming tips* to help you work on yourself from without as well as from within.

» Each day of the program ends with a Night Thought, something to help orient you positively for the next day—an idea, a lyric, a bit of poetry that will help you along the road to centering yourself emotionally and spiritually.

ONCE YOU'VE BEEN THROUGH THE 30-DAY PROGRAM YOU WILL NOT ONLY LOOK AND FEEL BORN AGAIN, YOU WILL HAVE CHANGED YOUR APPROACH TO LIVING. The amazing part is that all this will happen almost automatically, because the Born-Again phenomenon is experiential. You don't just read about it, you *live* it. And once having lived it, you're on your way to a new life . . . permanently. I know this because it happened to me, and I've seen it happen time and again to others. The results of the Born-Again Program will be external as well as internal. You'll be able to look in the mirror and love who you see.

THAT SPECIAL RADIANCE IS THE LOOK OF THE "BORN AGAIN." It's a gift that's there for the asking, for anyone, anytime, no matter what your age.

Come. Follow me.

CHAPTER 4

Secrets for Living Longer . . . and Better

The idea of being able to control how long we live has probably had its appeal since the human brain evolved to the point of being able to conceptualize something so wonderful.

The fact is that we *do* have a lot more control over both the quality and length of our lives than we think. The real question is whether we want to do what we have to do in order to exercise that power.

TO LIVE WELL AND LONG, YOUR APPROACH TO LIFE MUST BE BALANCED AND WHOLE, AND YOU MUST KNOW WHAT KINDS OF FOODS TO EAT AND IN WHAT PROPORTIONS. It's never too late to change. The story of my father-in-law, Harry Gross, is an example. At the age of sixty-three, Harry was suffering from arthritis, had kidney and lung problems, and was verging on a nervous breakdown.

For a long time Harry had been addicted to cigarettes and alcohol. His diet ran to fats and cholesterol—sour cream, lox, *kugel,* and cheese pie. Most of his friends ate the same way, so it didn't seem unusual to Harry. Nor did he give a thought to all the medicines he was taking for his various ailments. Most people in America *expect* that by the time they reach their sixties the whole mechanism is going to begin breaking down. Medicine becomes a way of life. Aches and pains become a way of life.

My husband, Bob, didn't see life this way at all. He was involved with the American Natural Hygiene Society, a group dedicated to healthful living through natural methods. Hygienists follow the lean, sensible diet now recommended by the latest nutritional research: high in natural, or complex carbohydrates, low in protein and fats. Bob begged his father to change his diet and the whole way he was living. It saddened him to see Harry wracked by arthritis and fits of coughing, and unable to work at the tavern he owned because his health was so poor.

Finally, Harry gave in. He went to a fasting institution to undertake a twenty-day fast. There he broke his old addictions, purged his system of its toxin build-up, and got his body to a state where it could respond to the new diet he would follow.

That fast, the first of many that Harry would undergo in the years to follow, marked the beginning of his new lease on life. Down the drain with the tranquilizers and medicines. He stopped smoking. He became the bane of his wife's existence by refusing her breads and well-marbled steaks. Eventually Sara went along with her husband's new eating plan and got a vegetable juicer for their kitchen. Still, she laughed at him when he got up early to exercise.

Instead of driving everywhere, Harry began walking. Though he was over sixty, Harry had made a choice. He'd decided to add years of usefulness, vigor, and health to his life. His reward? Another quarter of a century of the good life. Harry lived to be eighty-seven and he was free from the old aches and pains. Until the very end he functioned so well he was able to work part time (he'd sold the tavern and got into a healthier occupation), and drive from New Jersey to Hyde Park, New York, to visit his grandchildren.

FAY MORRIS WAS CHRONICALLY ILL AND ONLY FORTY-NINE YEARS OLD. Twenty-five years ago, at the age of forty-nine, Fay Morris of Toronto, Canada, was plagued with back and internal problems. She'd worn a spinal brace for two years and had been in and out of doctors' offices for longer than that. "I was low in body, mind, and spirit," Fay recalls. Then she discovered a health spa near Niagara Falls, New York. The spa's rejuvenation program included a week on nothing but water, to "eliminate the body poisons." Fay went home looking and feeling like a different person. She decided to give up her old way of living, to fast regularly, to stop eating refined, processed foods, and to make daily physical activity a part of her life.

As is so often the case, Fay had family resistance to cope with at first. Her children joked about "mother's eccentricities." But as Fay grew stronger, slimmer, and brimming with energy, the family changed its tune. Now her husband, Harvey, is as enthusiastic about fasting as she is.

For the past twenty-five years, Fay has taken her summer vacation at fasting retreats, fasting up to two weeks at a stretch. Besides fasting periodically, she adheres to a simple vegetarian diet that's mostly made up of raw foods. A jogging enthusiast, ten years ago, at the age of sixty-four, Fay achieved the honor of being the oldest person to finish a grueling 100-mile centennial run sponsored by Toronto's YM-YWHA. She accomplished this feat in five weeks, running in three-hour stretches. At the age of sixty-four! "I have more pep now than I did when I was in my thirties and forties," says this vibrant, youthful seventy-four-year-old.

HERE'S THE SIMPLE ROUTINE THAT KEEPS FAY LOOKING AND FEELING INCREDIBLY YOUNG.

- » She wakes up every morning at six, and, weather permitting, is off to a nearby track for a brisk hour-and-a-half walk.
- » Four mornings a week she eats nothing before going to her Health Club for a three-mile run, a calisthenics workout, and eight lengths in the pool!
- » Afterward she goes home for a light meal of fresh fruit and natural cheese, followed by a rest.
- » Mid-afternoon, Fay has her special "elixir," made by putting parsley, celery, carrots, and beets through her juicer.
- » For dinner she has a large raw green salad with a dressing of cold pressed oil. With it she has either a baked potato or cottage cheese. She never has coffee, tea, milk, or dessert.
- » Ordinarily she's in bed by 10:30 P.M.

SENATOR WILLIAM PROXMIRE LOOKS TEN YEARS YOUNGER THAN HE IS. At sixty-one, an age when most men in this country are already heavy-jowled, wrinkled, and pot-bellied, Senator Proxmire of Wisconsin looks and acts at least ten years younger. Proxmire, who jogs five miles from his home in Cleveland Park to his office in the Capitol daily, started running years ago. He's well known for his frugal eating habits. He proselytizes. One of his staff members is chided regularly for eating chocolate covered doughnuts in the office. The youthful looking senator is a public example of a man who's learned how to slow down the aging process.

There are a lot of books being written about how to live longer. They go into long, scientific explanations about cross-linkages and free radicals and the bonding of protein molecules and somatotypes and chromosomes. What it all boils down to is this. *If you cut down on the stresses and abuses you're inflicting on your cells, you'll slow down the aging process and add years to your life.* The people whose stories I've related became motivated to do just that. They and others like them have proved beyond doubt that no matter what weaknesses you were born with, you can stay younger longer, and even regain lost youth. All you have to do is make a decision about the way you're living.

Montaigne, the great philosopher, said, "Man does not die; he kills himself." Herbert Shelton, the father of modern rational fasting, puts it another way. "We are killed by the toxins we learn to tolerate." Dr. Hans Selye, the expert on stress, sums it up. "Every stress leaves an indelible scar," he says. "The organism pays for its survival after a stressful situation by becoming a little older."

THE NORMAL LIFESPAN OF HUMANS IS 100 YEARS OR MORE. Animals live on the average from five to seven times the length of time it takes them to reach maturity. There's no reason why humans shouldn't do as well. Assuming that the average human is mature at twenty, 100 to 140 should be *your* normal lifespan.

Children today mature faster and grow larger than children of past generations did. This may actually be due to an abnormal acceleration of the aging process. If the diet of rats is restricted during their early development to a level of food intake that is close to fasting but still sufficiently nutritious, the rate of maturation slows down and the rats live longer. Studies of humans conducted by the Dutch scientist, Dr. Fritz De Waard, establish a link between diet and the early onset of puberty. Dr. De Waard found that in countries where people can't afford to buy much meat, milk, eggs, and butter, girls begin to menstruate later than do those in more affluent countries. People in these "low cholesterol" countries do not grow as large; they also do not have as high an incidence of cancer and heart disease. Scientists are beginning to feel that this idea of raising each new generation to be "the biggest and the best" may be contributing to a speed-up of our life cycles as well as the premature occurrence of chronic diseases, old age, and death.

*   *   *

I SET BACK MY OWN TIME CLOCK. When I was twelve years old I got my first menstrual period. In those days I was gorging myself on all the contraband hotdogs, milkshakes, and pecan pie I could get my hands on. I was physically well developed for my age. By the time I was fourteen I was so mature looking that some mistook me for an older, married woman.

At the age of fifteen, after I'd started to fast occasionally and completely changed my eating habits in an effort to control my psoriasis, I stopped menstruating. Worried, my mother consulted Herbert Shelton, one of the early founders of therapeutic fasting. He explained to us that girls who follow a low-protein, natural carbohydrate diet tend to mature, physically, at a later age than others and often don't menstruate until their late teens. (I began menstruating again at nineteen.) The fact is, stressful living habits and poor diet will cause your cells to mature faster than they should. After changing to my new diet, I began looking younger. I've stuck to the natural carbohydrate diet ever since, and to this day I look younger than many my age. So does everyone who lives the way my family and I do.

Here's What to Do to Turn Back Your Time Clock

1) *Keep your protein intake level down.* Remember that according to new government reports (and also well-known nutritionists like Dr. Jean Mayer and Dr. Nathan Smith) it's possible to overdose on protein. Calculate your individual needs and control your PI (Protein Intake): (Chapter 5 will tell you how.)

2) *Raise your consumption of natural carbohydrates.* Carbohydrate metabolism is much less aging than protein metabolism.

3) *Remember that minimum is adequate.* Less food means more life, it's as simple as that. Too much of anything, even high quality food, causes more work—hence stress—for your cells.

4) *Cut out saturated fats.* These are real agers. Avoid them in meat, cheese, butter, hydrogenated oils, commercial peanut butter, and fried foods.

5) *Stick to live (not processed) foods.* You can't maintain vigorous life on a diet of dead foods—and that's just what white sugar, white flour, pastries, and most processed foods are: DEAD. *Natural* carbohydrates are the best source of energy.

6) *Learn to eat simply and only when hungry.* By eating fewer big

meals and by eating only one concentrated protein or one concentrated carbohydrate at any given meal you take a lot of stress off your digestive system. (See Chapter 8 for the rules of proper food combining.)

7) *Stop dumping drugs and chemicals into your system indiscriminately.* This includes coffee, tea, chocolate, preservatives, vitamin pills, tranquilizers, aspirin, sleeping pills, cocaine, marijuana, alcohol, amphetamines, cathartics, and laxatives. All of these things poison your cells and cause you to age before your time.

8) *Get the breath of life into your cells by exercising.* Walk. Run. Swim. Bicycle. Play tennis. Ski. Jump rope. Chop wood. Dance! Join an exercise class! Be active and learn to love it! Exercise is absolutely essential for optimum health and longer life. (Follow the exercise plan in Chapter 15.)

9) *Quit smoking.* Smoking is a life-quencher. It causes your skin to wrinkle prematurely. It decreases (seriously) your chance to live. It's the perfect insurance for death, not life.

10) *Learn the secret of your own happiness.* It will not only add years to your life but life to your years. Have worthwhile goals for your life. Earn your living by doing some kind of work you enjoy if you possibly can. Learn how to meet the challenges and setbacks and even griefs of your life with a positive attitude. Let each failure be a learning experience, a strengthening factor in your life. Find joy in seeking answers to problems. It will help your mind to grow and will lead you into happiness on a level you've never known.

11) *Rest.* It gives your cells a chance to regenerate. Your brain, nerve cells, digestive system—all of you needs this opportunity daily. Don't try to shortchange yourself. You'll only shorten your life and make it less relaxed and enjoyable.

Health, youth, and longer life are what this book is all about. It makes no difference how old you are at this very moment—you still have a choice to make. There's still time to be born again.

CHAPTER 5

The Dynamic New Natural Carbohydrate Diet

When my mother was in her mid-thirties she was introduced to the practices of a small but lively group of people who followed a way of life that kept them amazingly healthy and young looking. They called themselves Natural Hygienists. The organization still exists (it grows larger every year), and the people affiliated with it continue to enjoy the results of this remarkable, health-maintaining, anti-aging way of eating.

I CALL IT THE NATURAL CARBOHYDRATE DIET. It has kept me unusually healthy and young looking throughout my adult years, just as it did my mother. But the exciting news, and one of the reasons I decided to write this book, is that modern nutritionists have begun to recommend "new" dietary principles that are the very same as the ones my husband, my children, and I and many of our friends who are Natural Hygienists have lived by all our lives.

SCIENTISTS ARE NOW RECOMMENDING A DIET FAR LOWER IN PROTEIN AND FAR HIGHER IN NATURAL CARBOHYDRATES. They've found that too much protein isn't good for you and that most Americans eat two to five times more than they should. *Nutritionists now tell us that natural carbohydrates are the healthiest and least aging way to get energy.* In fact, the new U.S. Senate Committee on Nutrition and Human Needs recommends that natural carbohydrates make up 55 to 60 percent of your diet.

A certain, minimum amount of protein—10 to 15 percent—is

necessary and important for the functioning of the body, but as we shall see in this chapter, diets that are too high in protein contribute to weight problems and early aging.

The New Facts on Protein

Protein helps children build new tissues (growth) and helps adults repair tissues that are worn out and need replacement (maintenance). These two functions, growth and maintenance, are equally important but they require very different amounts of protein. *Because we were taught as children that we needed protein to make us grow, many of us continue to eat high quantities of protein as adults, thereby causing ourselves problems.*

Protein, the only nutrient to contain nitrogen as well as carbon, hydrogen, and oxygen, is made up of building blocks called amino acids.

It's the protein in muscle that allows it to contract and hold water. In hair, skin, and nails, the protein is hard and insoluble, providing the body's protective coating. Protein also helps build bones and teeth. Probably because protein *is* of basic importance in human nutrition, a number of myths and misconceptions have sprung up about it.

COMMON MYTHS ABOUT PROTEIN. One idea that persists is that many Americans are eating protein-deficient diets. Actually, there are very few of us who need more protein than we're getting. Most need less. "In the U.S., chances are small that any adult who is receiving a calorically adequate diet could be deficient in protein or in specific amino acids," says Dr. Jean Mayer, the outstanding nutritionist and president of Tufts Medical College.

There are really only three categories of people who are "protein vulnerable" and should watch to be sure they're getting enough. These are women who are pregnant or nursing, people who swing back and forth from one fad diet to another, and children who subsist mostly on dry cereal, soft drinks, and other processed or refined sugars and starches.

ANOTHER MYTH IS THAT PROTEIN IS OUR BEST SOURCE OF ENERGY. It isn't; natural carbohydrates are. Their work is to provide energy for the brain, muscles, and the central nervous system, while protein's work is tissue building and repair. If you rely on protein for *energy,* you can actually create a deficiency in which there's not enough protein left over to do its proper work.

TOO MUCH PROTEIN CAN HAVE AN AGING EFFECT ON HUMANS. Before the protein in meat can be put to use, it has to go through a process called deamination, in which the nitrogen is removed from the molecules. These are reconstituted in a form the body can use. At the same time, toxic by-products of animal protein—mainly urea and uric acid—have to be gotten rid of by the liver and kidneys.

The digestion of plant protein is much easier on the body (there's virtually no deamination and no toxic by-products to be gotten rid of), and the digestion of carbohydrates is easier still.

A diet that's too high in protein—especially complicated animal protein—can wear you down and age you prematurely.

WHEN YOU CONSUME MORE PROTEIN THAN YOUR BODY CAN ACTUALLY USE, YOU TEND TO PUT ON WEIGHT. That's right. Protein, like starch, has 4 calories per gram. After it's deaminated, some of the leftover residue gets turned into fat, and that fat is stored in your body. The more protein you eat, beyond what your body needs, the more fat you're likely to store from it.

HOW DO I KNOW HOW MANY GRAMS OF PROTEIN I'M CONSUMING? That's a good question. Most people haven't the vaguest notion of how much protein they actually eat.

You have been told by others to count calories. You have been told by others to count carbohydrates. But you have never been told by anyone to count protein. I'm telling you to count protein. You have to learn how to count it—every day, gram by gram, until, like counting calories, it becomes second nature. And it *will* become second nature. Eventually you'll know instinctively how much is just right for you. But first . . .

YOU'LL NEED A SPECIAL TOOL TO HELP YOU CONTROL YOUR PROTEIN INTAKE AND WORK OUT A NEW WAY OF EATING THAT WILL KEEP YOU AMAZINGLY SLIM AND VITAL. To control your Protein Intake there are three things you need to know.

» *First* is how many grams of protein your particular body needs each day to carry out its work of tissue building and repair.

» *Second* is how many grams of protein you're now actually consuming each day.

» *Third* is knowing the Protein Count (PC) of the various foods you eat so you can figure out your daily PI and then alter the amount you're now consuming accordingly.

REMEMBER, ANY EXCESS PROTEIN YOU CONSUME IS GOING TO MEAN EXTRA CALORIES AND PREMATURE AGING. It's that simple. If, for example, your body needs only 45 grams of protein a day and you're consuming 90, you are definitely overdosing on protein. The longer you continue to eat more protein than you need, the more likely your body will run down prematurely. For years now, people have labored under the delusion that they can eat as much protein food as they want and stay slim and healthy. *This is simply not true.* It's why so many are eating themselves fat, even though they're very conscientious about "sticking to protein."

WITH THE INFORMATION IN THE FOLLOWING TWO CHARTS, YOU WILL HAVE A BRAND-NEW FORM OF DIETARY CONTROL. Chart A will tell you what your Protein Intake *ought* to be. After you figure this out, you will then go to Chart B.

Chart B is a Protein Counter. With it, you can find out how much protein you're actually consuming each day. Subtract what you *should be* consuming (Chart A) from what you're *actually* consuming (Chart B) and you'll know how much you have to cut down.

Find yourself on this chart by looking first for your age category. There you will find listed the number of grams of protein per pound of body weight you need. *If you are an adult over the age of nineteen, the chart says you need .36 grams of protein per pound of your ideal (not actual) body weight.* Say your ideal body weight is 130. You multiply 130 by .36 and get an answer of 47, indicating that what you need is about 47 grams of protein a day.

If you're between the ages of fifteen and eighteen, your multiplier is .40. As you can see by the chart, the *younger* you are, the more protein you need.

(The body's need for protein remains fairly constant, but can vary as a result of certain stresses or demands. To be sure that people in stressful periods of their lives will get enough protein, *the Food and Nutrition Board recommends as a minimum requirement, twice what the*

CHART A

RECOMMENDED DIETARY ALLOWANCE FOR PROTEIN

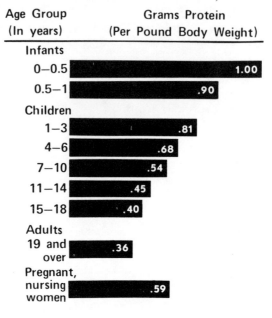

Age Group (In years)	Grams Protein (Per Pound Body Weight)
Infants	
0–0.5	1.00
0.5–1	.90
Children	
1–3	.81
4–6	.68
7–10	.54
11–14	.45
15–18	.40
Adults 19 and over	.36
Pregnant, nursing women	.59

average person needs. Bear this in mind when figuring out your own protein needs. If you're going to tamper with the figures, tamper on the low side, not on the high side.)

Chart B, which follows, is a sample Protein Counter based on data from the U.S. Department of Agriculture. (You will find a complete Protein Counter in Appendix C.)

This sample Protein Counter gives the measure of food, the amount of protein in grams, and the number of calories. Calories are included so you can see how some foods that are low in calories *could* make you gain weight, if you overeat them, because their protein count is so high. (Three ounces of crab meat is only 5 calories, but it's 9 grams of protein!)

Bearing in mind that most adults need no more than 30 or 40 grams of protein for their total daily intake, let your eye glance down the "Protein Grams" column of the following Sample Counter. Afterward, we'll discuss what some of this information means for you.

CHART B

YOUR SAMPLE PROTEIN COUNTER

(Note: These foods are listed for purposes of information and comparison only— NOT *because they're recommended for your New Lifetime Eating Program)*

MEAT AND FISH

Portion	Protein Grams	Calories
3 oz. lean beef (pot roasted)	23	245
3 oz. hamburger	23	185
3 oz. sirloin (broiled)	20	330
3 oz. beef (oven roasted)	17	375
½ chicken breast (fried)	26	160
3 oz. chicken (skinned, broiled)	21	120
1 cup canned chili (without beans)	19	340
3 oz. corned beef (canned)	22	185
1 lamb chop, 3.1 oz. (broiled)	18	360
1 pork chop, 2.7 oz.	19	305
2 oz. boiled ham (sliced)	10	130
1 frankfurter (boiled)	7	170
3 oz. bluefish (baked or broiled)	22	135
1 cup crab meat (canned)	24	135
3 oz. tuna (drained solids)	24	170
3 oz. swordfish (broiled)	24	150
3 oz. sardines (drained)	20	175
8 oz. (or 8) fish sticks (breaded, frozen)	40	400

EGGS AND DAIRY FOODS

	Protein Grams	Calories
1 egg (whole, raw)	6	80
1 cup cow's milk	8	150
1 cup milk (evaporated)	17	340
1 in. cube Cheddar (or American)	4	70
1 cup cottage cheese (creamed)	28	235
1 cup cottage cheese (uncreamed)	25	125
1 cup yogurt (partially skimmed)	12	145
1 oz. Swiss cheese	8	105

LEGUMES AND NUTS

	Protein Grams	Calories
1 cup red beans (canned)	15	230
1 cup split peas (dried, cooked)	16	230
1 cup lima beans (cooked)	16	260
1 tbsp. peanut butter	4	95

Portion	Protein Grams	Calories
½ cup peanuts (roasted, salted)	18.5	420
½ cup cashews (roasted)	12	392
½ cup almonds (shelled)	12	387
½ cup Brazil nuts	2	92

GRAINS AND GRAIN PRODUCTS

1 cup barley (uncooked)	16	700
1 cup cornmeal (dry)	11	435
1 cup rolled oats (cooked)	5	130
1 cup rolled wheat (cooked)	5	180
1 cup rice (cooked, long grain)	4	225
1 cup macaroni (cooked)	7	190
1 slice bread (whole wheat)	3	65
1 tbsp. wheat germ	2	25

FATS, OILS

1 tbsp. margarine	Trace	100
1 tbsp. corn oil	0	120
1 tbsp. cooking lard	0	115
1 tbsp. mayonnaise	Trace	100
1 tbsp. French dressing	Trace	65

VEGETABLES

1 cup asparagus (cooked spears)	3	30
1 cup green beans (cooked)	2	30
1 cup broccoli (cooked)	5	40
1 cup cabbage (raw, shredded)	1	15
1 ear sweet corn (cooked)	2	70
Boston lettuce (1 5-in. head)	2	25
Iceberg lettuce (1 6-in. head)	5	70
1 cup mushrooms (canned)	2	20
1 cup green peas (cooked)	8	150
1 potato (baked in peel)	4	145
1 cup spinach (cooked)	5	40
1 cup soybean sprouts (raw)	6	40
1 cup winter squash (baked)	4	130
1 tomato (raw)	1	25
1 cup turnip greens (briefly cooked)	3	30

FRUITS AND FRUIT PRODUCTS
(raw, except when noted)

Portion	Protein Grams	Calories
1 apple	Trace	80
3 apricots	1	55
½ California avocado	2.5	185
1 banana	1	100
½ cantaloupe	2	80
1 cup cherries	2	105
1 cup dates (dried)	4	490
3 figs	1	90
½ white grapefruit	1	45
1 cup grapes	1	65
1 orange	1	65
1 cup orange juice from frozen concentrate	2	120
1 cup papaya	1	55
1 peach	1	40
1 cup raisins	4	420
1 wedge watermelon	2	110

One idea that should jump out at you quickly after looking over the Protein Counter is this: *If you eat meat or fish once a day and sometimes more, you'll find it almost impossible NOT to eat too much protein.* If you're an adult whose ideal weight is 130 (and you're not ill, or pregnant, or nursing) then 47 grams of protein a day is adequate. Say your lunch is a salad made of 3 ounces of tuna (that's the very small can) and half a cup of cottage cheese. That's 38 whopping grams of protein right there! Now, top it off with just the smallest, leanest broiled steak for dinner (3 ounces), and that's another 20 grams. Already you've gone over your protein allowance by 11 grams.

Inevitably, of course, you'll end up consuming even more protein than that during the day, when you count the juice, or toast, or salad, or what have you. Almost everything you eat has *some* protein—except for pure fats and refined sugars.

Even people who don't eat meat can easily overdo when they're not aware of their body's real protein needs. It was long thought that the only way to be a vegetarian and be healthy was to load up on foods high in vegetable or plant protein. The latest research shows that if you rely heavily on grains, beans, and dairy products in the hope of getting *enough* protein, chances are good that you're going to get *too much.*

Say you're a vegetarian who should be getting about 43 grams of protein a day. For breakfast you have 1½ cups of oatmeal liberally sprinkled with wheat germ and doused with milk. A good, healthy, high-protein breakfast in the minds of many, but look how it costs out. You get 7.5 grams of protein in the oatmeal, 4.5 for ¼ cup of wheat germ, and 4.0 for ½ cup of milk. That high-protein breakfast is high, all right—16.0 grams worth!

For lunch you have open-faced toasted cheese sandwiches—two slices of whole-wheat bread, each with an ounce of Swiss cheese on it. Zap! That's another 24 grams right there, for a total Protein Intake, so far, of 40.0. For dinner all you need is a measly cup of cooked lima beans at 16 grams, and you're at 56.0—way over your daily allotment. Of course one day like that isn't going to hurt you, but take in that extra protein day after day, and you'll probably be gaining weight and wondering why.

IT'S EASY TO SEE THAT THE HEALTHFUL PROTEIN ALTERNATIVE FOR EVERYONE, VEGETARIAN OR NOT, IS TO GO HEAVY ON FRESH FRUITS AND VEGETABLES. With a diet high in these natural carbohydrates, you still get the protein you need. You keep your weight down and have high energy too!

There are many surprise pluses to a diet high in natural carbohydrates, but before we go into them, I'd like to divest you of one last myth about protein. *It's the idea that plant or vegetable protein is not as good for you—not as "complete"—as animal protein.*

"Complete" proteins are those made up of all eight of the essential amino acids. The essentials are so named because they're required for human nutrition but can't be manufactured or synthesized by the body fast enough to meet its needs. It's essential, then, that we get the balance of our amino acid requirements directly from the foods we eat.

All eight essential amino acids must be present in the body if any one of them is to do its work. Since many animal protein foods contain all eight of the essentials, nutritionists used to think that meat was necessary to a healthy diet.

WHEN YOU EAT A VARIED DIET OF VEGETABLE PROTEIN FOODS, INCLUDING PLENTY OF DARK, LEAFY GREEN VEGETABLES, YOU'LL GET THE BALANCE OF ESSENTIAL AMINO ACIDS THAT YOU NEED. In general, vegetable protein doesn't have the concentrated nitrogen that animal protein has (nitrogen is the trigger that activates growth and repair), but what it does have is more readily available for use in the body. Nutritionists now use the term "viability" to describe foods whose protein content can most easily be turned to good use by the body. Many vegetable protein foods are highly viable. Vegetable protein is "live," which means it will sprout or grow if exposed to proper conditions.

Vegetable protein is protein the way nature made it—in the plant. And the plant is where the animal first went for *its* protein.

The following foods are excellent sources of plant protein. Look them up in the comprehensive Protein Counter at the end of the book. And remember! Gram by gram, proteins add up more quickly than you think!

Almonds	Corn	Rolled oats
Asparagus	Fresh green peas	Romaine lettuce
Brazil nuts	Fresh sprouts	Sesame seeds
Broccoli	Kale	Soybeans
Brown rice	Lentils	Spinach
Cabbage	Lima beans	Turnip greens
Carrots	Okra	Whole rye
Cashews	Potatoes	Whole wheat
Collards	Pumpkin seeds	

Give special attention to the dark, green, leafy vegetables like romaine and spinach. These contain all the essential amino acids but one—methionine—and that can be gotten from eating small quantities of seeds or nuts.

MODERN TRAINING PROGRAMS FOR ATHLETES STRESS NATURAL CARBOHYDRATES. It used to be thought that the more you physically exerted yourself, the greater your need for protein. Modern nutritional studies have proved this untrue. Dr. Jean Mayer says, "Although the body does 'turn over' protein and needs regular replacements, it doesn't turn it over a bit faster whether you're an Olympic swimmer or just an ordinary citizen who sits and watches the Olympics on TV."

Some of the country's most famous athletic coaches and marathon runners have discovered that *a diet made up predominantly of natural carbohydrates provides almost three times the strength for endurance in athletic competition than a diet high in protein and low in carbohydrates.*

There's a reason for this. Protein has to be converted into carbohydrate before it can provide the body with energy. The rate of conversion just doesn't keep up with the athlete's rate of energy expenditure.

Carbohydrates, requiring no such conversion, give *direct* energy. Some of them, such as fruit, are so simple in structure they require virtually no digestion, being absorbed into the bloodstream directly from the stomach. For this reason, natural fruit juices are now used widely to give athletes the quick, lasting energy they need.

The New Facts About Carbohydrates

At the beginning of the century, almost 40 percent of our caloric intake in this country came from *unrefined* carbohydrates: fruit, vegetables, and grain products. Today, little more than 20 percent does. This is because our fat and refined sugar consumption has risen out of all proportion to what's good for us.

Last year every man, woman, and child in this country consumed 125 pounds of fat and 100 pounds of sugar—statistics uncovered by the U.S. Senate's Select Committee on Nutrition and Human Needs. Soft drink consumption is up to 275 cans a year per capita—a "formidable quantity," as Senator McGovern, head of the Committee, puts it.

In setting up new dietary goals for the U.S., the Senate Committee recommended a dramatic boost in the level of carbohydrate and natural or fruit sugar consumption—up to over 50 percent of the total caloric intake.

OVER HALF THE PEOPLE IN THE WORLD STAY THIN ON A NATURAL CARBOHYDRATE DIET. This is because they eat primarily low-density, or watery, carbohydrates—fruits and vegetables whose fiber creates filling bulk, but whose caloric and protein count are low.

Carbohydrates—made of carbon, hydrogen, and oxygen in the proportion seen in water—are also major sources of energy for most of the world's people. They are produced in green plants by the light from the sun working on carbon dioxide and water.

Carbohydrates come to us as starches and sugars for nourishment, and as cellulose for roughage or fiber. Virtually every kind of fruit falls into this category, as well as whole grain foods and starches, such as brown rice, millet, and corn. (Vegetables are really neutral, but since they do contain starchy cellulose, I include them when I speak of natural carbohydrates.)

In a normal diet, it's the *natural* carbohydrates that constitute the principal supply of energy. The diet prevalent in America today, in which fats and refined sugars are supplying more energy than natural carbohydrates, is abnormal.

A WORD ABOUT CARBOHYDRATES AND JUNK FOOD. Junk foods give carbohydrates a bad name. Candy, honey, jellies, molasses, syrups, soft drinks, and other sweets processed from sucrose, or table sugar, contain little if any nourishment. The same is true of cakes, cookies, and breads processed from refined white flour. These are called "empty calories" because, indeed, they contribute nothing but calories to the diet.

Why Natural Carbohydrates Make You Feel Good and Look Good

Here are some reasons why natural carbohydrates are vital to good health, low weight, and super energy.

1) *Natural carbohydrates provide direct energy for the brain, muscles, and body tissue.* They convert easily to glucose, a type of natural sugar that's the body's main source of energy. This conversion to glucose is the main point of carbohydrate digestion.

Carbohydrates are protein-sparing. They quickly and efficiently provide the energy your brain and muscles need, while leaving the protein's energy for its proper work of building and repair.

2) *Natural carbohydrates, when varied and plentiful, will provide enough protein to meet your daily dietary needs.* That's right. Carbohydrate foods also contain protein, and a diet high in natural carbohydrates is protein safe, as you'll quickly see when you begin using your Protein Counter.

I rely mainly on fresh fruits, vegetables, seeds, and a minimum of grain, and I get all the protein I need. I avoid milk and eggs and eat only moderate amounts of cheese, because of the high fat and cholesterol content of these foods. I eat whole grain foods— steamed brown rice, corn, an occasional slice of whole grain bread, etc.—but I watch the amounts because I've found that starchy foods tend to get you into the syndrome of "the more you eat, the more you want."

The thing to understand is this. You don't really have to worry about protein as long as your diet is high in *natural* carbohydrates and low or (ideally) absent in refined ones.

3) *Natural carbohydrates are not fattening.* Any reputation carbohydrates have for being fattening comes from the "junk" or refined carbohydrates. When you compare *natural* carbohydrates with foods high in protein—especially complex animal protein—you'll find that, on the whole, carbohydrates rate lower in calories. The Senate Committee suggests that the best way "to ease the problem of weight control" is to eat more natural carbohydrates. "The high water content and bulk of fruits and vegetables and the bulk of whole grain can bring a longer lasting satisfaction of appetite more quickly than do foods high in fats and refined processed sugars."

4) *Natural carbohydrates give you the vitamins and minerals you need.* The report issued by Senator McGovern's Committee also pointed out that "increased consumption of fruit, vegetables and whole grains is important for an adequate supply of micronutrients, vitamins and minerals in the diet."

Dr. Jean Mayer and Dr. Nathan J. Smith, the expert in sports medicine, agree that when your diet is well balanced and high in natural carbohydrates, you'll have all the vitamins you need—right from nature.

5) *Natural carbohydrates put all-important fiber in your diet.* Cellulose, the residue of the digestion of fruits, vegetables, and whole grains, provides the fiber necessary for normal, healthy bowel action. (Low-fiber diets, such as those high in animal protein, have been shown to contribute to all kinds of chronic bowel trouble, including colitis and cancer.)

6) *Natural carbohydrates help maintain the proper water balance in your bloodstream.* Fresh ripe fruits and tender young vegetables are high in water content, and water is the medium in which all the chemical reactions in your cells take place. Sixty percent of your body weight and 90 percent of your blood plasma is water. This water carries the salts and proteins so important in nutrition.

7) *Natural carbohydrates power the heart.* The heart is a muscle and muscles need glucose, the fuel supplied by carbohydrates. There's evidence that diets high in natural carbohydrates may reduce the risk of heart disease. *Most population groups with the lowest incidence of coronary heart disease consume very high quantities of carbohydrate—from 65 to 85 percent of their total caloric intake.*

8) *Natural carbohydrates feed your central nervous system.* While mus-

cles, in a pinch, can draw on stored reserves of glucose, the central nervous system can't. It needs a continual, minute-by-minute supply. As I've said, the foods that provide glucose most directly are natural carbohydrates.

9) *Natural carbohydrates are the healthiest and most satisfying way to take care of a "sweet tooth."* Ten calories of fructose (fruit sugar) is 50 percent sweeter than the same amount of table sugar. What better way than sun-ripened fruits to satisfy the craving for something sweet?

10) *Natural carbohydrates cut down disease and premature aging.* By boosting your carbohydrate consumption you'll be cutting down on fats, refined sugars, and protein, of which the vast majority of Americans eat far too much for optimum health and longevity. Carbohydrate metabolism is the easiest by far for the body to tolerate, and it throws off no toxic by-products. *Eat MORE carbohydrates and LESS protein and you can actually do something positive and direct to keep yourself younger, healthier, slimmer, and more vital.*

It has been proved to me time and time again that the simple, natural way of life works. I saw it first in my mother, then in my own life, and finally in the lives of literally thousands of others, many of whom I've met in various regional chapters of the Natural Hygiene Society, and many, many more who've come to our own Pawling Health Manor over the years. What we've all found is indescribable joy in this natural way of life, this natural diet. Indeed, it provides the basis for a true "natural high"—one that is always with you, one that gives you the energy and enthusiasm you need for an active, busy, vital life.

Turn in your old diet and sedentary regime. The euphoria of health can be yours!

CHAPTER 6

A New Solution
for the Overweight

Last year, Dr. William E. Connor of the University of Iowa told the Senate Select Committee on Nutrition and Human Needs that the vast majority of Americans suffer from an overabundance of food contributing to such illnesses as coronary heart disease, high blood pressure, diabetes mellitus, and obesity. He and other scientists have incriminated not only *how much* you eat, but also *the kinds* of foods you eat. They tell us that a diet high in calories, saturated fats, salt and sugar, low in fruits and vegetables, and distorted by a high intake of processed foods is a diet that contributes significantly to a wide range of health problems.

People with chronic obesity often get panicked as they watch the pointer rising on the bathroom scale. That panic or feeling of desperation can make you run to artificial means for help. Let's have a quick look at some of these artifical means and see what they do to us.

Amphetamines, known colloquially as "speed," act on the hypothalmus in such a way as to deaden the appetite. They also stimulate the central nervous system and are seriously addictive. In recent years the FDA has set up stricter rules governing their use, and while they're not as indiscriminately prescribed as they used to be, many overweight people still manage to get and depend on them for appetite control.

Diuretics are often prescribed by doctors for weight loss. People who are overweight have excess fluid trapped in their fatty tissues. These fluids can result from using too much salt and other spices, but instead of restricting their patients' intake of salt and seasonings, doctors will often put them on diuretics. Diuretics will cause you to loose fluid, temporarily, but they'll also stimulate the loss of certain vital minerals, such as potassium, that have to be replaced with more pills. People on diuretics can easily find themselves involved in a cycle of pill-taking that can be hard to break.

THE PROTEIN-SPARING "FAST" CAN BE DANGEROUS. You're given a jug of artificially colored liquid made from animal collagen, synthetic vitamins, and enough water to make the stuff pour. It sells for up to $80 a bottle and is worth $4.50, according to the Food and Drug Administration. You're instructed to have 300 or 400 calories worth of this pink goo daily, plus all the diet soda, coffee, and tea you want.

Some people refer to this diet as a fast. It is *not* a fast. Any nutrient at all that you take into your body will trigger action in the digestive system and create a need for the *entire spectrum* of nutritional components. This is known, biochemically, as the All or None Law. On the protein-sparing diet you're not getting any carbohydrate and you're not getting any fiber, but you are getting protein, vitamins, and other chemicals. At the same time you're permitted stressful ingredients in the form of artificial sweeteners, dyes, and chemicals in the no-cal drinks, and the caffeine in tea and coffee.

To neutralize the imbalance created by these toxic substances the liver must work abnormally hard. It must also break down the protein for energy. The fats released as a result of this breakdown are turned into glucose by means of the tricarboxylic cycle. This contributes to the already acidic condition in your body. It can lead to a dangerous state of acidosis and renal shutdown, in which the kidneys, overworked by the need to excrete abnormally large amounts of urea and uric acid, simply quit.

THERE'S A HEALTHY WAY TO TAKE OFF WEIGHT FAST AND KEEP IT OFF. If you need to lose a lot of weight and want the psychological boost that rapid weight loss can give you before you begin a new and lifelong plan of proper eating, *true fasting* is a far better way to do it. In a true fast the body has nothing at all to digest, so it does not go into a state of nutritional imbalance. Rather, it goes into a state of total physiological rest. A special fasting metabolism takes over (See Chapter 7) that allows the body to live off its own fat reserves.

Here are the stories of four people who finally got their weight problem in hand through the method I describe in this book.

JACK JOHNSON, AN INSURANCE EXECUTIVE FROM BALTIMORE, MARYLAND, WAS PLAYING A DANGEROUS GAME WITH HIS LIFE. During his thirties his weight had risen slowly but without interruption until now, at the age of forty-one, he tipped the scales at 215. Most of his excess weight was distributed more or less evenly over his five foot ten inch frame, but his belly protruded as sharply as a pregnant woman's. His blotchy, ruddy face mirrored a blood pressure reading of 160 over 120.

When I first met Jack, after he arrived at the Manor to begin a fast, he was literally afraid for his life. He would groan as he eased himself into a chair. His hands trembled as he reached for his water glass on the bedside table. Breath tinged with the odor of stale garlic, vodka, and nicotine permeated the room.

"A few weeks ago," he recalled, "I thought I'd pulled a muscle in my leg because it had turned black and blue. I went to my doctor and he told me I'd ruptured a main blood vessel. Soon I developed other, smaller ruptures in my buttocks. The bruises were a sign of subcutaneous hemorrhaging. The doctor told me to quit smoking and drinking and to cut out coffee. 'Otherwise,' he said, 'your next visit to me will be for treatment of heart attack—if you survive it, that is.' To tell you the truth, Mrs. Gross, I was afraid to tell the doctor about the pains I'd started having in my chest."

Under careful supervision, Jack went on a Total Water Fast for eighteen days and then spent three days gradually breaking his fast on fresh juices. At the end of the fast he'd lost twenty-eight pounds, his hands were steady, and his facial tics and nervous twitches were gone. He was cautioned that a fast is only the beginning of the road to health, that a return to smoking, drinking, and poor eating habits would surely bring back the dangerous symptoms he'd arrived with. Then we gave him the precise information he'd need for his new, lifetime eating plan—the same one I lay out for you in this book.

SOL FELDMAN HAD BEEN OVERWEIGHT SO LONG HIS WIFE HAD LOST INTEREST IN HIM. So far all of Sol's attempts to get back to his normal weight had failed. "I tried everything," he told us, when he arrived for his first fast. "Pills, shots, hypnosis, high-protein—you name it, I tried it. The trouble is, I would always lose some, and then gain it right back again. This time I'm going to get it off and keep it off!'"

As his marriage disintegrated Sol had put all his efforts into becoming a successful businessman. Now he could afford the best of everything, including the handsome Porsche which was parked out front—but neither his expensive possessions nor his fine clothing could glamorize the 300-pound mass of his flesh.

Sol came to us determined to change his life through fasting and I'm happy to tell you he won the battle. During the year following his first visit to the Manor he lost over a hundred pounds! He set himself a goal and eventually, through periodic fasts and careful monitoring of the quantity and quality of the food he ate, he reached it. Although, like any of us, he would backslide from time to time, his real determination never faltered. As he lost pounds, he regained his self-respect. "For years," Sol told me recently, "all I'd ever heard from my wife was, 'Don't, Sol, you'll mess up my hair,' or, 'Sorry, I've just put on lipstick.' Now that I've lost all this weight my wife actually feels possessive of me. She respects me. We've developed a new, exciting relationship."

BILL SMITH WAS THE SURPRISE VICTIM OF "CREEPING OBESITY." "Something happened to my body in the summer of 1973," he wrote, after I'd asked him to describe his experience. "An illness had me grounded for six weeks and I put on weight. Instead of shucking it after my recovery, I watched in horror as the scales approached 240 pounds! Sure I'm six one, but ordinarily my weight didn't exceed 210. This excess weight I couldn't get rid of was slowing me down, even making me depressed. My doctor prescribed medication for my high blood pressure, high blood sugar and for gout, but with that and dieting as carefully as I could, I only lost a little and my blood pressure was still on the rise.

"A friend at the office dropped a book about fasting on my desk one day and proceeded to inform me about something I'd never heard of before—therapeutic fasting. I was doubtful, but curious enough to discuss it with my doctor. 'Don't go,' was his advice.

"I decided to go anyway. Taking several books with me as well as a radio and a shopping bag full of medicine, I checked into the fasting institution on January 4, 1976.

"By seven o'clock that night I was as hungry as I'd ever been, but things began to go better the next day. I found that what I'd heard was true. The hunger feelings go away very quickly on a fast.

"On my second day I drew a huge grid chart to track my weight loss. At the end of ten days the curve on my chart resembled a satisfyingly steep flight of descending stairs.

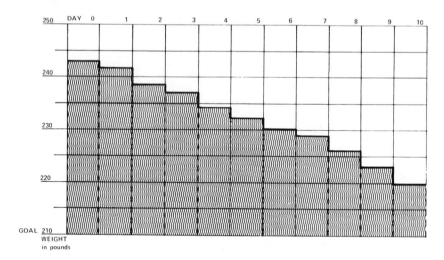

"Almost twenty-three pounds in ten days! That's something no diet can do! At 220 I felt better than I had in years. Fasting had really done something for me beyond taking off the pounds. In the hope of getting my weight down to my optimum 210, I made plans for another fast in the spring. I returned on April 11 for a one-week stay and lost not ten more pounds but fourteen! (Incidentally, the bag of pills I'd carried with me on my first trip is still untouched. I find it scary to think that if it hadn't been for my fasting experience I might still be popping those things at the rate of ten a day.)"

ONLY TWENTY-THREE, SUSAN PATTERFIELD WAS THIRTY POUNDS OVERWEIGHT AND SUFFERING FROM HYPOGLYCEMIA AND CONSTIPATION. Her physician had put her on several kinds of medication, including diuretics, but things weren't getting any better. Desperately unhappy, Susan decided to try a fast.

Hers was a case that responded well to short, regular fasts of several days' duration. With a strict eating plan in between fasts, along with careful withdrawal from the drugs she'd been on, Susan lost twenty-five pounds and regained her feelings of health and energy.

Several weeks after she returned home she wrote me this letter, which she has given me permission to share with you.

DEAR JOY,

I feel wonderful! I haven't felt this good in years. I can't tell you how different it is to finally be off all that medication. I have so much energy. Before I was draggy and tired constantly. The big surprise is that my bowels have been working by themselves for the first time in two years.

There's another surprise, too. Recently Jeff and I went for a climb at Monument Mountain and I brought along raw vegetables for myself and a couple of sandwiches for him. Lo and behold, when he saw all the vegetables he passed up the sandwiches and started eating *my* lunch. Now he's begun changing his eating habits and asking all kinds of questions about what's good for you and what isn't. I feel so much better physically and mentally. I can't adequately express to you how I feel and how my experience has changed my life.

SINCERELY,
SUSAN

The stories go on and on. Not a week passes that someone doesn't report a complete turnabout in life to me. Just recently I was finishing up my weekly lecture on nutrition at the Manor. "Have any of you found *any* method of weight reduction that's successful in keeping off the weight once you've lost it?" I asked the guests.

An attractive, dark-haired woman at the back of the room raised her hand. "I was here a year ago," she replied. "When I checked in I weighed 230 pounds. I fasted for seven days and lost fourteen. Then I went home and made all those changes in my eating habits you'd told me about. I lost another eighty-six pounds, for a total of 100, and now I'm here working on the last ten."

As you might imagine, everyone in the room applauded. Joan Mansfield had changed so drastically in looks and demeanor both that I hadn't even recognized her!

THE METHOD JOAN USED TO GET THIN AND STAY THIN IS THE SAME METHOD I'M SHARING WITH YOU IN THIS BOOK. It's the same new way of life which helped me to overcome my psoriasis. It's the same new way that helped Sol and John lose weight and regain their health and sexual vitality. It's the same way of life that Dr. Jack Goldstein talks about in his book, *Triumph Over Disease*. In describing his long, healing fast, Jack wrote: "I was destined to make a decision that was to change the entire course of my life, the lives of my wife and children, and the lives of thousands of people with whom I would cross paths. I was going to hang onto precious life. I was not aware of it at the time, but I was, in a sense, going to be REBORN. . . .”

THROUGH RATIONAL FASTING, YOU, TOO, CAN BE REBORN. The following chapter will tell you how you can fast at home for short periods, or where you can go away for longer, supervised fasts. Fasting may be the break you need to help get you off your food addictions, but as the stories above show, it is not in itself the cure for obesity. You have to change your whole approach to eating and living. By supplying your body with good, natural foods and the right emotional and physical environment, you can create a new you, one that's young, beautiful, and happy.

WHAT ELSE YOU CAN DO IF YOU'RE OVERWEIGHT. Get yourself a calorie counter. Learn the caloric value of the foods you eat. You'll be shocked by what you're consuming.

Here's a breakdown, by calories, of the sort of lunch that's popular among teenagers and business people alike.

Three ounces of roast beef contain 375 calories. The bun (or two slices of bread) costs another 120 calories. Add 70 to 100 calories for mayonnaise. That amounts to 595 calories for the sandwich alone.

Chances are you won't stop with the sandwich. If you have an eight-ounce milk shake (281 calories), ten french fries (57 calories), and one chocolate chip cookie (104 calories), you have totted up a horrendous 1,047 calories for just one meal!

If you're five feet four inches and want to keep your weight at about 110 pounds, say, your total caloric intake per day can't exceed 1300 calories. If you're not physically active, then 1200 calories a day would be more realistic.

Assuming you're fairly active and can maintain your weight loss on 1300 calories a day, the roast beef lunch has left you with only a 250-calorie allotment for breakfast and dinner both.

You'd be wiser to think like this: I can have a whole grapefruit for 80 calories, with ¼ cup of sunflower seeds for 175 calories, costing me a total of 265 calories for a super-nutritious breakfast.

For lunch I can have a lucious fruit salad (10 large strawberries, ½ cup fresh pineapple, ½ cup fresh papaya, a sliced orange, and a scoop of cottage cheese) for a total of 310 calories. For dessert, a cup of herb tea with lemon will cost me nothing. So far I've spent 575 calories for two meals (less than the one roast beef sandwich we were talking about), and I still have 725 calories left for the day.

There are some who would tell you that at this point you're free to "splurge" those 725 calories on steak with béarnaise sauce for dinner. Not I! The point of this whole book, remember, is not simply to teach you how to keep your weight down. It's to teach you how to live abundantly while eating to achieve maximum energy and to keep your body from wearing down and aging before its time. So forget about the "splurges." All that stuff is bad for you! Eat light and also eat right!

For dinner, then, you can have (for example) a huge green salad using ½ pound of romaine lettuce, 10 mushrooms, ½ a cucumber, a ripe tomato, 10 sprigs of watercress, and ½ a green pepper. (Total so far: 126 calories.) You can have a dressing made with 1 tablespoon of cold pressed oil (120 calories), lemon juice (only a trace), and a pinch of Vegebase (25 calories), bringing the count for salad and dressing up to 271. Eight spears of asparagus will cost you 20 calories, a large baked potato with a pat of butter, 136 (100 for the potato, 36 for the butter). The total meal comes to only 427 calories.

With 298 calories left over, your whole day's meals will have cost you fewer calories than the roast beef sandwich, milkshake, french fry, and cookie meal. You can save your extra calories in your calorie bank, or use them for a snack before bed, or add them onto your evening meal.

THERE'S MAGIC IN PERSISTENCE. Once you've decided to think for yourself it will get easier. Learn how to eat and live so as to be the beautiful person you were designed to be. Only you can make that beautiful, healthy you a reality. It all depends on how successfully you resist such destructive influences as the ice cream store, the bakery, the pizza parlor.

The magic lies in resisting temptation and sticking to your new, life-giving regime. YOU CAN DO IT!

CHAPTER 7

Fasting to Look Younger (and Lose Weight)

A lot has been said about fasting as a method of weight loss, and indeed you can lose weight quickly this way. But to me what's even more exciting about fasting is its rejuvenating effect. Fasting will give your system a total physiological rest and allow it to clean out cellular debris or stored-up toxic materials. If you fast periodically you can actually end up looking younger. Herbert Shelton, now in his eighties, has supervised the fasts of over 50,000 people during the last half century at his fasting institute in San Antonio, Texas. In his book, *Fasting Can Save Your Life,* he says:

Anyone experienced with fasting has seen many instances of physical rejuvenation—stepped-up vigor, increased mental powers, loss of weight, greatly increased functional vigor, with better digestion and bowel action, clear sparkling eyes, clearing of the complexion with a restoration of youthful bloom, the disappearance of some of the finer lines of the face, reduced blood pressure, better heart action, sexual rejuvenation. Fasting can bring about a virtual rebirth, a revitalization of the organism. As the fast progresses, all of the cells of the body undergo refinement and there is a removal from the protoplasm of the cells' stored foreign substances so that the cells become more youthful and function more efficiently.

If that isn't a selling testimony on the benefits of fasting, I don't know what is. I use Shelton's words because he's had such vast experience helping people to rejuvenate themselves through fasting, but I can tell you from my own experience as well that incorporating short fasts into your life can make an enormous difference in how you look and feel. It will help you break your addictions to destructive, acid-forming foods and it will prepare your body to respond optimally to the fresh, natural carbohydrates you're going to be eating more of on your new Lifetime Eating Plan. Fasting is the most efficient way to make the switchover from your old way of life to the new one that's going to bring such marvelous changes. There is also, as we shall see, scientific evidence of its remarkable rejuvenating powers.

PEOPLE HAVE KNOWN ABOUT THE BENEFITS OF FASTING FOR A LONG TIME. Fasting has been practiced for various reasons from early recorded history. The Bible tells us that Jesus fasted for forty days and forty nights. Ghandi used fasting as a penance and as a means of political protest. In more recent times civil rights leaders such as Martin Luther King, Jr., Dick Gregory, and Caesar Chavez have used fasting both for spiritual reasons and as protest measures.

It wasn't until the early nineteenth century, however, that physicians and others began to document the physical benefits to be reaped from going without foods for extended periods of time. In 1823 a young Amherst college graduate and Presbyterian minister, Sylvester Graham, began to champion the cause of Natural Hygiene. After studying physiology in an attempt to improve his own ill health, Graham became a brilliant lecturer and writer and started the natural health movement in America. "Graham" bread and "graham" crackers took their name from him. He advocated vegetarianism and fasting. Russell T. Trall, of New York, Isaac Jennings of Connecticut, Thomas Low Nichols of Boston, and William A. Alcott (uncle of Louisa May Alcott) were physicians of that time who gave up practicing orthodox medicine and built their practices around Graham's principles of fasting and food reform. Dr. Trall opened the first Hygienic Institute, in New York City, in 1847. His first patients were a group of desperate cases from Broadway Hospital, all of whom recovered.

In the beginning of the twentieth century, Dr. Linda Burfield Hazzard wrote a book called *Fasting for the Cure of Disease,* in which she presented dramatic, fully documented case histories from her own practice.

At about the same time, fasting was further brought to public attention by novelist Upton Sinclair, who regained his broken health by fasting and wrote a book about his experience, called *The Fasting Cure.*

SCIENTIFIC STUDIES ON FASTING AND REJUVENATION HAVE BROUGHT FORTH SOME FASCINATING MATERIAL. Professor C. M. Child of the University of Chicago did research on aging in animals for more than fifteen years. He discovered that certain species of insects with access to abundant food pass through an entire life cycle in three or four weeks, but when their food is cut back and they're forced to fast periodically, they continue young and active for three years and more. Child's conclusion was that "partial starvation (fasting) inhibits senescence. The starveling is brought back from an advanced age to the beginning of postembryonic life; it is almost reborn."

The experiments of the noted French scientist, Dr. Alexis Carrell, author of *Man, the Unknown,* showed that waste materials and toxins are what cause cells to age. Dr. Carrell kept fragments of a chicken heart alive for many years. He found that they aged when not kept free of their own cell wastes—in other words when their own metabolic waste was allowed to remain in the culture medium in which the parts of the heart were kept.

What a Fast Can Do for You

CELLS GO THROUGH THE SAME LIFE PROCESSES YOU DO. They nourish themselves, grow, reproduce, respire, excrete. And there's something else. They can heal and rejuvenate themselves. That means that if you provide the right environment for your cells, you'll be rejuvenating your body.

There are two interrelated processes that go on inside you continually: anabolism and catabolism. Anabolism is the process of building up body tissues with nutrients. Catabolism is the breakdown of nutrients to release energy so that anabolism can occur. A fast expedites anabolism, or the building and repairing action within your cells. It also helps the cells do a better job of throwing out accumulated waste, since the body that's on a fast doesn't have to expend energy digesting and absorbing food.

Fasting is not in and of itself a "cure." What it does is allow the body the complete physiological rest it needs so that the organism can then become more efficient in healing itself.

Fasting will bring your body new power for flushing out toxic matter and poisons that have been accumulating inside you for years. It will improve circulation and give you new vigor, endurance, and stamina.

WHEN PROPERLY MANAGED, FASTING IS AN EFFECTIVE AND SAFE WAY TO LOSE WEIGHT, REGAIN A HIGHER LEVEL OF HEALTH, AND REJUVENATE YOUR BODY CELLS. Scientific studies show that humans not only survive but can radically benefit from rational, lengthy fasts. (Note: Long fasts should *always* be supervised and conducted at a fasting institution.)

A few years ago two physiologists from M.I.T., Vernon R. Young and Nevin Scrimshaw, presented fascinating documentation to the scientific community proving that a forty-day fast is well within the capacity of the normal, healthy adult. In an article in *Scientific American* they pointed out that recent tests of total fasting for weight reduction have yielded remarkable results. Obese individuals have gone without food for extended periods of time and have emerged from their experience in good health and many pounds lighter. "From a purely biochemical standpoint," they wrote, "the most efficient way to lose weight is complete fasting into the stage where body fat is being consumed as the main source of energy for the brain and other tissues."

How Fasting Works

As you settle into a fast, your system mobilizes itself for survival. Its primary need is for glucose to supply energy for the vital functions. Your brain is the most critical user of this fuel. Two-thirds of your body's total circulating supply of glucose goes to the brain; the rest goes to muscles and red blood cells.

In order to provide your brain with glucose when you haven't eaten for several hours, your liver begins to draw on the fatty tissues in your body to synthesize what it needs.

DURING A FAST YOUR BODY GOES INTO A SPECIAL FASTING METABOLISM THAT PREVENTS YOUR VITAL TISSUES FROM BEING USED. Your body begins to break down stored fat cells and use as fuel a substance that gets released during the breakdown: *acetoacetic acid.*

This breaks down further into substances called *ketones*. When oxidized, ketones produce energy. This process is called *ketosis*. On a long fast (one that continues for a week or more—the sort that should be conducted only at a fasting institution), the brain begins to rely on ketosis for most of its fuel for energy. So does the rest of the body. (A helpful side effect of the ketosis state is that you lose your appetite!)

FASTING IS NOT STARVING. You may fear that if you miss three meals in a row your vital tissues are in danger of breaking down. They're not. Ample scientific evidence proves that before reaching a starvation state you'd first have to use up all your stored nutritive reserves—glucose, bone marrow, extraneous fat. Not until all your reserves run out—usually after some thirty to fifty days—would your body begin to break down its vital tissues. On a properly supervised fast you would never be allowed to continue long enough to approach the starvation phase. The crucial distinction is this: in fasting you're being nourished on stored surpluses. In starving you're living on vital tissue and will ultimately die if you persist. Instances of death from self-imposed starvation are extremely rare.

How to Manage a Short, Safe Fast at Home

Many people have begun fasting themselves at home for several days at a time. It's like putting yourself on a miniature de-tox program. You get off the coffee, cigarettes, alcohol. You break patterns of overeating. Just like breaking a drug habit, you can break the habit of "needing" salt, spicy foods, soft drinks. You can wean yourself from that special category of foods I call "addicting" because they tend to make you want to eat more and more of them. Many of the addicting foods are processed grains: breads, cereals, and pasta.

While long fasts at specially supervised fasting institutions are the ones generally thought of as therapeutic, you can do yourself a lot of good by taking short fasts from time to time.

Studies of the short, intermittent fasting of mice, conducted by Clive McKay, of Cornell University, are considered classics in the physiology of fasting. Comparing a control group that were fed all they wanted with a group of mice fed sparingly on a high-quality diet and fasted frequently, McKay found that the latter developed more slowly but were healthier and lived *five times longer* than the control group.

Depending upon the health and weight problems of the given individual, people have reported all kinds of improvement as a result of fasting for brief periods at home.

H.K., a secretary, writes:

I've not only maintained the twenty-five pound loss I achieved during my two-week stay at Pawling Health Manor but by following your carbohydrate regimen and fasting one or two days, at intervals, I lost nearly ten pounds more. I feel 100 percent better and my friends tell me I look at least ten years younger . . .

I.M., a business executive writes:

I want to thank you for re-educating me and prolonging my life. I left the Manor at 178 pounds (a twenty-two-pound loss in two weeks) and have maintained my loss by staying on my new eating regimen. This week I fasted four days at home and lost an additional five pounds. Fantastic! Not only that, my blood pressure, which used to be way up, has dropped to normal. My doctor is very pleased with what I've done for myself.

FASTING SHOULD NOT BE TAKEN LIGHTLY. Three or four days is long enough to fast at home, unsupervised. If you have diabetes, heart disease, conditions like ulcerative colitis, or epilepsy, or if you're on medication like dilantin, diuretics, tranquilizers or lithium, you need special supervision and should check with your physician before beginning a fast.

PSYCHING YOURSELF UP TO BEGIN. There are several things you can do to help you get past your last reservation and take the plunge. First, look in the mirror. You can erase some of those lines, get rid of that second chin (if you have one), flatten out that stomach. To psyche yourself into your first fast you have to want these things and you also have to believe that if you fast intermittently and follow the Natural Carbohydrate Diet between fasts, they *will* happen! You can get rid of minor aches and illnesses, headaches, fatigue. You can have, instead, new, super energy and a more youthful appearance. You can *feel* younger and you can live longer when you begin to care for yourself in this new way. Remember that mini-fasts are as important a part of health as is eating healthfully. I do it myself once or twice a year. Mini-fasting is part of our family's way of life. Don't let anyone frighten or discourage you. This can be a first step forward toward a born-again you. Plan now to set aside three or four days for fasting, as soon as possible. To further your inspiration, read *Therapeutic Fasting,* by Arnold Di Vries, and *Fasting Can Save Your Life,* by Herbert Shelton.

HERE ARE SOME THINGS YOU SHOULD KNOW BEFORE STARTING A SHORT FAST AT HOME.

1) *What to drink and when to drink it.*

Drink only fresh, pure water when fasting, and drink only when thirsty. You can't "flush out your system" by drinking huge amounts of water, so don't try.

Spring water is best. Buy a gallon of spring or distilled water before you begin. It will more than last for your three-day fast.

Cool water is best, although during cold weather people sometimes find hot water comforting. Or, you may want a little crushed ice sometimes. Just be sure it's made with distilled water and that you chew it thoroughly so that it melts before you swallow it.

2) *Things that may happen to you during a fast.*

You may have a *headache* for a few hours at the beginning of your fast, or you may suffer some *nausea* or even throw up. (Shelton says that vomiting may occur in one out of ten persons during a fast.) In any event, don't worry about these symptoms. They are only an indication that your body is housecleaning. It's like kicking a drug habit. You're kicking the food-and-stimulant habit.

Dizziness may occur from time to time, although if you understand why it's happening you can take steps to avoid it. During a fast, a definite physiological slowdown occurs as your organs adjust themselves to a reduction in nutritive supplies. The heart rests and the rate of circulation slows down. There's less blood in the brain (although thinking is clear). If you start up quickly from a sitting or prone position, you could experience dizziness or faintness. To avoid this, simply take care to rise or sit up slowly, so that the circulation of blood in the brain has a chance to adjust.

Sometimes you might experience a feeling of fear or unsureness or notice that your heart is beating too fast. *Lie down.* These symptoms indicate that your glucose reserves are being used up, that you're using more fuel than is available. Rest, then, is essential to cut down on energy consumption. If the symptoms persist, don't hesitate to break your fast with an orange or a grapefruit. This should restore your feeling of well-being and allow you to resume fasting.

3) *Smoking, drinking, and drugs or stimulants are out!*

The worst thing you could do to yourself, during a fast, is take toxins into your systems. If you are on any sort of medication requiring careful withdrawal, have your physician tell you how to manage this before you begin your fast.

WHAT YOU MAY AND MAY NOT DO DURING A FAST.

Exercise squanders your glucose reserve so I don't advise exercising while fasting. It uses energy your body needs for its rest and repair. Particularly strenuous activity such as sports, heavy outdoor work, or heavy housecleaning could make you feel dizzy or faint. When animals hibernate—a practice that resembles fasting—they stop all activity and sleep. Even if your main goal in fasting is weight loss rather than rejuvenation, you'll get the best results if you curl up, keep warm, and concentrate on rest and relaxation.

Baths and showers are fine, so long as you don't make them enervating experiences. Tepid water—water close to the natural body temperature—is the least taxing to the organism.

Saunas or steam baths are not a good idea. They cause the body to expel large quantities of water, but not waste. Actually, they are an artificial means of trying to force the body to excrete waste through the pores and by flushing water through the kidneys. In fact, that's all that happens. Sweating and drinking, the person flushes water through his body, but no waste, bile, or urea is eliminated this way. Forced sweating is a stress situation that's not good for the faster.

Sunbathing, in moderation, can be a pleasant way for you to reduce tension while fasting. On the other hand, if you sunbathe for excessively long periods, or when the weather's too hot, you are putting your body in a stress situation that isn't good for it.

Enemas have become popular in some areas of the country. The idea, once again, is that you're getting rid of horrible wastes. Wrong! You may be cleaning waste from your intestine, but that will happen anyway. And an enema will *not* get the toxins out of your blood. Detoxification is one of the things we're aiming for, and fasting is the most efficient and unforced way of achieving it. By fasting regularly and eating properly you will succeed in detoxifying your entire system!

How to Manage a Three-Day Fast, How to Break It, and How to Return to a Healthful Eating Program

DAY ONE (FRIDAY)

It's better to fast when you don't have to go to work. If you can't get a few days off, plan to start your fast on a Friday morning. You will find that during the first day or two of a fast you'll have enough left over glucose in your system to give you ample energy for work.

At night you will find yourself going to sleep with a comfortable, lighter feeling, having consumed nothing all day but pure water.

Sleep habits often change during a fast. You may find yourself sleeping more or less than usual. This is par for the course.

DAY TWO (SATURDAY)

When you get up in the morning step on the scale and notice the two-pound weight loss! Your eyes will be clear and rested looking. Your skin may even be smoother!

During a fast your entire digestive tract is at rest. This includes your large intestine, where feces normally accumulate. Probably your bowel won't move at all during a short fast. If you should have some diarrhea it means your system is trying to get rid of something toxic.

Keep warm and pleasantly quiet today. And remember, nothing but water when you're thirsty—no coffee, no tea (herbal or otherwise), no no-cal. *Nothing except water.*

If you're ordinarily a heavy coffee drinker you may have a headachey feeling in the morning. This is actually a symptom of withdrawal from caffeine! Some fasters find that when they return to food, they have no desire to return to caffeine.

Avoid the kitchen! The smell and sight of food—even an unpeeled orange—can present a great temptation, especially on a short fast like this where you're not really fasting long enough to enter the state of ketosis, which depresses the appetite.

If you live alone, clear out of the way everything edible that might tempt you. If you must prepare food for your family while you're fasting just try to enjoy the vicarious pleasure of your culinary activities, but with sealed lips! *No* tasting.

DAY THREE (SUNDAY)

Again, rest, keep warm, and don't exercise. Think of your fast as a complete pampering experience. Books, music, television, the crossword puzzle, whatever amuses you, as long as it's restful and not overly stimulating.

In the evening—three full days since your last meal, on Thursday night—you'll be ready to break your fast. If you've never fasted before it will be difficult for you to imagine the genuine pleasure you'll get when you have that first sip of fresh orange juice.

Twice before going to bed, have three ounces of freshly squeezed orange juice. It's a good idea to dilute this with two parts of water. (We call it three-and-two.) Or, if you prefer, you may have a whole orange or a whole grapefruit. If melon is in season a small piece of watermelon would be fine.

The way you return to eating is just as important and potentially beneficial as the fast itself. I am going to give you two plans for re-feeding after your fast. *The Stay-at-Home Re-feeding Plan* gives you an extra day of light feeding, which will allow your system a bit more time to complete its housecleaning and—if weight reduction is your goal—to lose an extra pound or two. Use it if you have time to continue an easy schedule.

The Back-to-Work Re-feeding Plan is for those who must get back to a job or other commitments, or who don't want to stretch out the re-feeding regimen. *With either of these plans you'll continue to reap the healthful benefits begun by your fast.*

STAY-AT-HOME RE-FEEDING PLAN

MONDAY MORNING:

Have either a 5 or 6 oz. glass of freshly squeezed orange juice
or
a small piece of ripe watermelon
or
a whole grapefruit or an orange
or
half a ripe cantaloupe, or honeydew, or Spanish melon.

MONDAY NOON:

Either two oranges or a whole grapefruit
or

melon again
>   *or*
one or two ripe tomatoes.
>   *or*
Put a couple of tomatoes in the blender with a stalk of celery and eat and savour with a soupspoon, like a frappé.
>   *or*
Top, peel and section a ripe, fresh Hawaiian pineapple. Feed half the pineapple, in sections, into your juice extractor. Sip this luscious nectar slowly. You can make this a special event by pouring the pineapple nectar into a chilled, tall-stemmed glass.

MONDAY DINNER:
Pick an item from either the breakfast or lunch selections.

TUESDAY MORNING:
Skip breakfast.
>   *or*
Have a grapefruit, or an orange or two, or a piece of melon.
>   *or*
Have an 8 oz. glass of celery, parsley, and carrot juice, made in your juice extractor
>   *or*
a ripe papaya
>   *or*
two ripe peaches.

TUESDAY LUNCH:
Finger Salad (see the Monday Back-to-Work lunch) with a cup of cottage cheese or 2 ounces of sunflower seeds.

TUESDAY DINNER:
Large tossed salad with alfalfa sprouts and ripe tomato sections
>   *and*
steamed summer squash
>   *and*
a baked potato (if you must have butter, skimp on it).

BACK-TO-WORK RE-FEEDING PLAN

MONDAY BREAKFAST:
Same as for Stay-at-Home plan.

MONDAY LUNCH:
Same as for Stay-at-Home plan.
>   *or*

Finger Salad: Several large leaves of romaine lettuce, celery sticks, green pepper slices, a large, ripe tomato, and a cup of cottage cheese.
or
If it's cold weather, have a ten-ounce serving of steaming vegetable soup (see recipe chapter), and some raw celery sticks.
or
A medium-sized tossed salad with dark green lettuce (you can mix Bibb and romaine), cucumber slices, tomato wedges, slivers of green pepper or other tender raw vegetable, and one cup of cottage cheese.
or
A fruit medley of fresh pineapple chunks, blueberries and strawberries (or any other fresh, juicy fruit in season). Top with a scoop of cottage cheese or plain yogurt, and garnish with *one* chopped English walnut, pecan, or a few sunflower seeds.
If you're taking lunch to work, you can take your own ripe tomato and other raw vegetables, with a small container of cottage cheese. Fruit is easy to pack. Instead of the cottage cheese you may, if you wish, take two or three ounces of raw nuts or seeds.

MONDAY DINNER:
Finger Salad (same as lunch)
and
ten steamed asparagus spears and a large baked potato.
or
Fruit Plate: mango (or peach slices) and pineapple sections arranged on a bed of crisp greens, sprinkled generously with large fresh blueberries and seedless white grapes. With this, a cup of cottage cheese *or* 2 or 3 ounces of raw nuts or seeds.

On Tuesday of the Back-to-Work Re-feeding Plan you would return to the principles of your Lifetime Eating Program as described in Chapter 8.

YOUR NEW LIFETIME EATING PLAN

Your New Lifetime Eating Plan

A recent government report says changes in the average diet in the U.S. since the beginning of the century may be just as profoundly damaging to the nation's health as the contagious diseases that were on the rampage in the early 1900s. The report blames the destructive dietary changes on the increasing affluence in our society. Isn't it ironic? Higher incomes have taken us away from what's good for us—diets high in greens, beans, and whole grains—and toward harmful diets filled with a lot of rich, fatty meat, refined and processed foods, and junk foods.

We don't have to give up our higher incomes, but we do have to rethink our attitudes toward health and get back to basics as far as our eating and living habits are concerned.

IT'S JUST AS EASY TO BECOME ENSLAVED TO GOOD HABITS AS TO BAD ONES. The purpose of this book is to help you take the plunge and begin enslaving yourself to good habits. Just as enslavement to bad habits causes your cells to sicken, age, and die prematurely, so enslavement to good habits can change your life for the better, physically, mentally, and even spiritually.

BREAK WITH THE PAST. The eating plan described in this and the following three chapters is not designed to remind you of your childhood feasts or your mother's tender proddings to EAT! My hope is that you'll forget most of your past associations with food and instigate brand-new ones that are based on newly proven scientific principles.

THE PLAN YOU'RE ABOUT TO EMBARK ON WILL FORM THE BASIS FOR AN EATING PATTERN TO FOLLOW THE REST OF YOUR LIFE. It's the same plan that's successfully used in Natural Hygienic institutions in the United States and Europe and which has brought improved health to countless thousands.

THERE ARE FOUR THINGS YOU SHOULD KNOW ABOUT YOUR NEW EATING PLAN.

It will make you look better—slimmer, smooth-skinned, bright-eyed. If you want to, you can lose between ten and twenty pounds in 30 days, as you will see when you follow the Born-Again Body Program at the end of this book. (It will help you put into practice everything you learn about eating in these chapters.)

It will make you feel better—healthier, more vital and super energetic. Because it's a low-salt, low-saturated fat, low-protein way of eating, it will lessen your susceptibility to heart disease, cancer, diabetes, skin problems, hypertension, and digestive difficulties.

It will cost you less money—many are finding that the high cost of meat plays havoc with the food budget. While prime quality fruits and vegetables aren't cheap—and they will be the mainstay of your new Eating Plan—they don't a hold a candle, in cost, to the price of meat.

It will save you time—simple, natural foods require less preparation. In fact, to get the most out of them you should cook them as little as possible. My "waterless" steaming method suffices, and it will cut your meal preparation time down to fifteen minutes. (See Chapter 11.)

YOUR PRIMARY GOAL ON THIS EATING PLAN IS TO GET TO THE POINT WHERE YOU'RE EATING ONLY THE HIGHEST QUALITY FOODS IN MINIMUM AMOUNTS. Remember, *minimum* is adequate! You can put that slogan on your refrigerator door, over your mirror, above your bathroom scale.

You may feel that it's too difficult to switch over all at once to your new, ideal diet. That's okay. You can break in gradually if you wish, switching first to the foods that appeal to you the most and gradually adding the others. It may take a while for your digestive system to become accustomed to handling these new "live" foods anyway.

Rational fasting is a good way of getting your body ready to begin your new Lifetime Eating Plan. Just a couple of days' fasting (as per the guidelines in Chapter 7), and you will suddenly appreciate the wonderful, natural flavors of unseasoned foods.

ALWAYS KEEP IN MIND YOUR GOAL—THE NEW, THINNER, HEALTHIER, BETTER-LOOKING YOU. Feeling better and looking marvelous will quickly compensate for the loss of acquired (and, therefore, expendable) taste thrills of past favorites like fried chicken, white bread, ice cream, and potato chips. You'll find yourself looking forward to more healthful pleasures—the taste of ripe mangoes, sweet, juicy grapes, a crisp green salad, baked yams.

LEARN TO THINK IN TERMS OF WHOLE FOODS. It's when you begin fragmenting foods by cutting, cooking, and preserving them that your system starts getting into trouble. Whenever you're able, eat your foods whole, just the way they grow in nature. Remember that nature has prepared them perfectly, complete with vitamins, minerals, enzymes, amino acids, natural sugars, fibers and water, in all the right proportions for efficient use by your body. Fresh, ripe fruits, vegetables, nuts, and seeds—carefully selected and prepared to suit your particular needs—are the super foods for the Born-Again Body.

THIRTY YEARS AGO I WAS A CLOSET VEGETARIAN. I can remember being seventeen and being teased by my boyfriend, Jimmy, when he found out about me. I was not only a vegetarian, but a natural foodist.

At first I felt odd about being different, but as I matured I quit worrying about what other people would think. More than anything I wanted to have smooth skin, and I was determined to overcome a serious condition that was interfering with my life. Cutting out the animal fats and excess protein was one of the things that helped.

As the years passed, I read and studied more on the subject of health and nutrition. I completely lost any desire I ever had for flesh foods. I also became attracted to a philosophy of life once expressed by Mahatma Ghandi: *"The only way to live is to live and let live.*" For me, this meant that the slaughtering of other animals is not within our rightful province.

It's been thirty-five years now since I've eaten meat, poultry, or fish. And my children have never eaten it at all! When scoffers try to argue with me about the nutritional adequacy of a diet that includes no flesh foods, I remind them that my children have grown up healthy. They've not only had far fewer illnesses than their peers but they're vigorous, energetic, and beautiful as well.

It may not be as easy for you to give up meat-eating as it was for me; I had a powerful motivation. For some people it takes time before new habits can be initiated. The 30-day menu plan I include in this book is a guide; it's the ideal toward which you can work. But if you find that vegetarianism is too much change for you to handle, there's an alternative plan that shows you how to incorporate fish and eggs into your meal plan as you make a sensible transition into the New Natural Carbohydrate Diet.

AS YOU BEGIN TO ORGANIZE YOURSELF FOR CHANGE, HERE ARE SOME VITAL POINTS TO KEEP IN MIND:

» Vegetarianism is more conducive to health and longevity than a diet that includes meat.

» Cultivating simple eating habits makes life easier, less expensive, and healthier.

» Chemical additives are dangerous. Stay away from foods that contain them.

» The average American eats twenty-five times the amount of salt he needs. Evidence shows a strong link between salt intake and high blood pressure. Eliminate as much salt and salty foods from your body as you can.

» Don't drink with your meals. Fluids dilute the gastric juices, rendering them less effective. They also tend to wash food through the digestive tract before it can be fully digested.

» Learn the science of food combining, as described in the following section. The way you feel and your health in general depends a lot upon how you combine your foods at mealtime.

» Take pride in being the mistress or master of your body. It requires courage to start being your own adviser. Change may be difficult, but the rewards are worth it. Think ahead to the satisfaction and excitement you'll feel as you begin looking and feeling better, happier, more vibrant because *you* are instituting changes in your own life.

FOOD COMBINING CHART

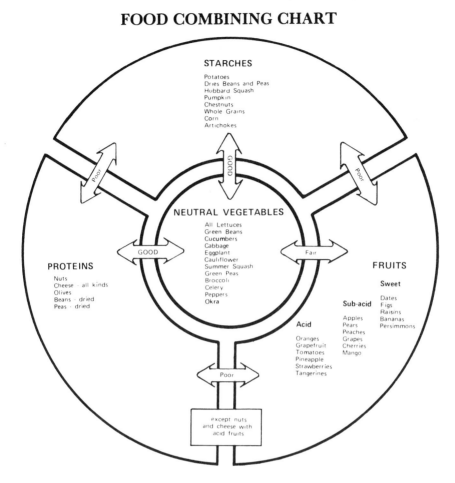

Avocados combine well with all foods except proteins and melons.
Tomatoes are best eaten with neutral vegetables and protein.
Melons are best eaten alone.

The Science of Food Combining

Basically, the idea of food combining is that different kinds of
foods, whether protein or starch, fat or acid, sweet or alkaline, require specific kinds of enzymes for their digestion. When you mix
foods together at one meal that call for opposite kinds of enzymic
action you interfere with their proper digestion.

Working with thousands of patients who've attended his Health School in San Antonio, Texas, during the last half a century, Dr. Herbert Shelton found that foods digest more easily when combined in a way that's biochemically harmonious. Based on principles first discovered by Professor Anton J. Carlson at the University of Chicago, Dr. Shelton established some significant rules of food combining. As I mentioned, my mother knew Dr. Shelton, so I began absorbing his rules years ago and follow them to this day. When you use these principles you will improve your general physical condition because the work of the digestive tract is made so much easier. You will also lengthen your lifespan. But if you're among those with chronic digestive problems, you'll have more to gain than anyone in mastering these principles. I have seen miraculous changes occur in the lives of people with colitis, diverticulosis, gall bladder problems, peptic ulcers, and acid indigestion, once they learned what food combining is all about and changed their way of eating accordingly.

At first the principles I'm about to outline for you may seem a bit complicated. However, once you begin following some of the menus at the end of this chapter, and after you complete the Born-Again Body Program, you automatically will have started to incorporate the science of proper food combining into your way of life. It's like learning a new language. You learn a lot faster when you go to the foreign country and begin speaking the language than you do just studying the textbook. So read through the following material with the idea of getting the basic gist of food combining. Don't become nervous that you won't remember it all. Just focus on the general underlying ideas. Remember that for 30 days you'll actually be living these ideas when you're on the Born-Again Body Program. After that, I guarantee all of this will seem quite simple—like speaking French after you've lived in France for a year.

1) *Eat only one concentrated food at a meal.* A concentrated food is one that doesn't have much water in it and is "dense," or high in calories—for example, grains, meat, cheese, fish, nuts, and seeds. You don't want to mix, say, meat and eggs, or cheese and nuts, or eggs and milk at one meal. Why? Proteins of different strengths and composition call for different digestive secretions as well as an entirely different timing of the release of secretions in order to be digested well.

Here are the basic concentrated protein foods:

Avocado	Eggs	Lentils	Nuts
Cheese	Fish	Meat	Poultry
Dried beans	Grains	Milk	Soybeans
Dried peas			

(*Note:* Avocado is a fat, and peas and beans are starches, but these are among those foods whose protein content is so viable or usable [half an avocado, for example, has as much usable protein as a glass of milk] that they should be considered for their protein value as well.)

2) *Don't eat proteins and starches at the same time.* You shouldn't, for example, have cheese at the same time that you eat bread, or meat at the same time you have potatoes. The reason? The stomach secretes a different kind of juice when you eat a starch food than what it secretes when you eat a protein food. In fact, starches and proteins require opposite media—starch requiring an alkaline medium, protein requiring an acid medium in which to digest.

Here are the basic starch foods:

Corn	Lima beans
Dried beans	Potatoes
Dried peas	Pumpkin
Grains (rice, wheat, rye, millet)	The winter squashes

3) *Eat acids and starches at separate meals.* Don't, for example, drink orange juice at the same time you eat toast. If you love orange juice when you get up in the morning, wait fifteen to thirty minutes before having a starchy breakfast of toast or cereal. The reason is that even weak acids destroy ptyalin, the enzyme that's necessary for the digestion of starches.

These are acid foods:

Grapefruits	Sour apples	Sour peaches
Lemons	Sour cherries	Strawberries
Limes	Sour grapes	Tomatoes
Oranges		

4) *Eat fats and proteins at separate meals.* Don't, for example, have ice cream for dessert after you've eaten steak. It slows down the digestion of the steak. So does a lot of oily dressing on your salad if you're having cheese with it. The reason is this: fat has a depressing

effect on gastric secretion. Since most proteins contain fat of their own, it takes long enough for them to be digested, without being held up further by additional fat.

Here are the basic fats:

Avocado	Nut butters	Seed oils
Butter	Nut oils	Shortening
Cream	Nuts	Tahini
Margarine	Olive oil	Vegetable oil
Meats		

(*Note:* Fat-marbled meats are better thought of as fats because their protein content doesn't compensate for the harm caused by their fat content. *Even the leanest meats that have had all visible fat trimmed off still contain 12 to 15 percent fat.*)

5) *Sugars and proteins should be eaten at separate meals.* Don't, for example, have bananas and cheese at the same time, or raisins and nuts. The reason is this: sugars undergo no digestion at all in the mouth or stomach, but pass right through to the intestine and are digested there. When you eat them with proteins or starches or fats, the sugars are held up in the stomach waiting for the other foods to be digested. While waiting, they begin to ferment. The digestive problems that result can cause gas, sour stomach, and bad breath.

Here are the basic naturally occurring sugars:

Bananas	Figs	Persimmon
Cantaloupe	Fruits (all dried)	Raisins
Casaba melon	Fruits (all fresh)	Sugar cane
Dates	Honeydew	Watermelon

(*Note:* Naturally occurring sugars are those found in nature—mainly fructose and glucose. They are to be distinguished from processed or refined sugars such as sucrose.)

6) *Starches and sugars should be eaten at separate meals.* Don't, for example, eat bread with jam, or pancakes with syrup, or cereal with sugar. The reason is this: starch digestion begins in the mouth and is completed in the stomach. Sugars, as I noted above, aren't digested in either the mouth or the stomach, but in the small intes-

tine. When you eat starch along with sugar, the same thing happens that happens when you eat protein along with sugar—the sugar gets held up in the stomach while waiting for the starch to be digested and fermentation sets in.

As you can see from these rules, the idea is not to "balance" a meal. Traditionally we've been taught to mix up everything at a meal—a little starch, a little carbohydrate, a little fat, and a lot of protein at every meal. No. This is overwhelming to the digestive system. No other animal in nature does all that mixing, including those whose digestive tracts are fundamentally the same as ours. The basic idea is to eat a concentrated protein food at one meal, and carbohydrates—either starches or sugars—at the next.

This does *not* mean, however, that you are only permitted one item of food per meal. There's another neutral category of foods. These are the succulent vegetables. Neutral foods are neither starch nor protein; at a meal they help to balance out either a concentrated protein food or a concentrated carbohydrate food.

The *green* succulents, especially, are important to the daily diet. They provide water, vitamins, minerals and amino acids, as well as the bulk you need for good digestion.

These are neutral foods:

Asparagus	Eggplant	Spinach
Broccoli	Green beans	Summer squash
Brussels sprouts	Kale	Swiss chard
Cauliflower	Lettuce	Watercress
Celery	Parsley	Turnip greens
Collards	Peppers	Turnips

Now, so you get the total picture, here are two days' worth of menus for properly combined meals.

SPRING AND SUMMER MENU

BREAKFAST	LUNCH	DINNER
Cantaloupe	Vegetable salad	Vegetable salad
	Okra	Broccoli
	Green squash	Fresh corn
	Jerusalem artichokes	Avocado

FALL AND WINTER MENU

BREAKFAST	LUNCH	DINNER
Persimmons	Vegetable salad	Vegetable salad
Pear	Kale	Brussels sprouts
Grapes	Cauliflower	String beans
	Yams	Pecans

I know that when you first look at menus like these they'll probably seem strange to you, but once you've begun eating this way, your body will tell you the wisdom of it. It's reasonable to assume that primitive humans didn't throw together all the different concoctions of food that we do and call it a meal. We were *meant* to eat simply. If you don't believe it just try combining your foods properly and see how you feel after a week or so. No more bloat, gaseousness, or twinges of heartburn and other signs of indigestion.

THE MONO-MEAL RESPITE. Every few weeks and sometimes more frequently, I follow the Mono-meal plan and eat only one item of food at each meal for a day. I happen to enjoy doing this with fruit, myself, but if you have any special digestive problems you'd be better off using the succulents, lightly steamed. Once you've been on your New Lifetime Eating Plan for several months and have completely corrected your digestive problems, you, too, should easily be able to handle a day of fruit.

I find that a day of Mono-meals is a good way to give my digestive system a rest, since I'm only eating one type of food at a meal and my enzymes and gastric juices need only do a minimum of work. I'll go to the market and pick out two or three kinds of the best looking, most tempting fruits I see. In the fall, when Tokay grapes are at their best, I'll buy several pounds of them, making sure the ones I select are dark red and ripe. When local peaches are in season I'll buy them a peck at a time, carefully selecting those that are darkest in color and firm, but not hard. The melons are good Mono-meal choices too—Spanish melon, or cantaloupe, or watermelon, in season. I've even chosen ripe bananas. In the case of oranges and grapefruits, I'll usually test, first, to make sure they're ripe and sweet. (For more information on how to select prime fruits and vegetables, see Chapter 11.)

The eating plan for the day is simple. I'll have nothing but one kind of fruit at a meal, and all that I want of it. For lunch I may have oranges—four or five of them if I'm so inclined. For dinner I'll have as many grapes as I want, two pounds if I feel like it. Actually, it's amazing how much pleasure you can get from eating simply in this way. No other flavors or textures interfere or compete with the particular taste delights of the fruit you choose. You could compare Mono-meal eating to decorating a room. When you clutter up a room with too many objects, no matter how costly or beautiful they may be, you can't fully appreciate any one of the objects as much as if it were in simpler surroundings. I will often have a Mono-meal for breakfast, one for lunch, and a large green salad and nothing else for dinner. Obviously this is not a plan to follow on a daily basis, but it's a good rest and recharger, especially if you've gone astray with your eating, as we all do, from time to time.

EATING SIMPLY HELPS TO MAKE YOU BEAUTIFUL. Way Bandy, make-up expert and beauty adviser to Elizabeth Taylor, Lauren Hutton, Joan Kennedy, Lee Radziwill, Diane Von Furstenberg, and other beautiful people, is a staunch advocate of the Mono-meal plan. Way, a glowing example of the Born-Again Body philosophy, believes that nutrition is the key to beautiful skin, "the sort you don't have to disguise," he says, "but can simply decorate." Way knows about food combining and warns his clients against toxic combinations. "Forget eating starch with protein. Eat one thing at a time—the mixture is what causes all the putrefaction," he says.

His own diet consists of live, whole fruits and vegetables, a diet from which he never deviates.

THE DIFFERENCE BETWEEN APPETITE AND HUNGER. An important part of following your new Eating Plan is learning to recognize the difference between appetite and hunger. Hunger occurs when your body cells have a genuine need for food to carry on the life process. To the hungry person some lettuce leaves or an orange can seem like a feast for a king.

Appetite, on the other hand, is false hunger. It's the body's craving for highly spiced foods, colas, coffee, and other irritants and stimulants to which your stomach is probably accustomed. When you first change your way of eating you'll probably feel those uncomfortable, gnawing sensations that occur when appetite demands satisfaction. Ignore these sensations and in a few days they'll be gone.

Appetite also occurs in relation to time. Most of us believe we need to eat at a certain hour every day. We've actually been brainwashed into expecting that something bad will happen if we don't have dinner by seven o'clock in the evening, or breakfast by eight in the morning. Yet skip breakfast entirely for a week and you'll find your early morning sensations of appetite have vanished.

It's important to begin ignoring the uncomfortable demands of appetite if you want to get onto a new and more healthful eating regimen, otherwise you'll never know when you're really hungry and will continue to be pushed around by cravings for highly stimulating, unhealthy, or empty foods. People with chronic problems of overweight will usually complain, "But I'm hungry." These people haven't the vaguest idea what true hunger is. Their bodies cry out to be fed five, six, seven times a day because they—the people themselves—have accustomed their poor stomachs to this abuse.

To get off the appetite kick, to reprogram your eating habits and return your body to its pure, natural state, you will have to suffer some withdrawal symptoms for a while, it's true. But these annoying symptoms won't last long *if your mental attitude is positive* . . . if you truly believe that you're not depriving yourself, but, far from it, are giving your body the first real gift it's had in a long time . . . if you can project yourself into the future a bit and imagine a time when you need only eat twice a day and yet be bursting with health . . . when you no longer salivate at the thought of french fries or a milkshake because you finally are turned on only by the foods that actually are good for you—then you will find those craving sensations last no more than a week, or even a day or two.

Not long ago the newspapers carried a story about a group of earthquake survivors who acted as if they were "going crazy" because they hadn't eaten in seventy-two hours. The article reported all sorts of bizarre behavior and attributed it to hunger. A man who'd been fasting with us at the Manor when this story appeared in the newspapers laughed out loud when he read it. "Look at this," he said to the other fasters. "I haven't had a thing to eat in seventy-two hours and I feel great and here these people believe they're going crazy."

It may be that the New Lifetime Eating Plan will seem abstemious to you at first, but you will soon grow to love it because you'll thrive on it. You can no longer think of the way you've *been* eating as normal. It's not. It's *abnormal.* You are going to retrain yourself to eat the way we human beings were meant to eat by nature, and when you do, you'll look back at your old eating patterns in amazement, wondering how you could ever have done that to yourself!

CHAPTER 9

Drinking and Health

Your body is approximately 60 to 70 percent water. Approximately 20 percent of this water is outside your cells, in your blood plasma, lymph, and connective tissues mainly. Approximately 50 percent is inside your cells. Your blood plasma is about 90 percent water. It's ultraimportant to supply your system with the water it needs on a daily basis.

YOU HAVE TO HAVE WATER IN YOUR SYSTEM IN A DEFINITE RATIO AND PROPORTION. When you don't have the right proportion of water in your blood plasma, cells, or interstitial fluid (that's the fluid that's outside your cells, in which they're "bathed"), your brain signals the pituitary gland, which releases an antidiuretic hormone, ADH, to control the water balance in your system. When there's too little water the brain signals the kidneys to reabsorb more filtered water back into your bloodstream. When there's too much water in your system, less water is reabsorbed back into your bloodstream. When your water balance is normal this signaling service isn't needed and energy is saved all around.

POTATO CHIPS, PRETZELS, PEANUT BUTTER CUPS, HOTDOGS, AND BALONEY SANDWICHES ROB YOUR SYSTEM OF WATER. When you eat mostly concentrated, refined foods—foods lacking in natural water—as so many Americans do today, you're reducing the water level in your bloodstream. Salty foods also reduce the water level, because salt absorbs water.

The soft-drink industry is booming because of this trend of eating relatively waterless, spicy, salty, concentrated foods—foods like gravies, bread, candy, ice cream, cake, pie, and pizza. This kind of unbalanced diet creates an omnipresent, almost insatiable thirst. Too often you turn to sugary drinks, sodas, and chemically loaded no-cals.

THREE REASONS WHY SOFT DRINKS AREN'T GOOD FOR YOU.

1) Regular soda contains refined white sugar—a dead food which leaches vitamins and minerals from your tissues and leads to vitamin deficiencies and tooth decay.

2) The chemical in soft drinks that acts as a flavor and color stabilizer is phosphoric acid. Phosphoric acid is fluid retentive, causes bloating, and has no place in your system.

3) Soda drinks contain coal-tar colorings. While red dye #2 and red dye #4 have been banned, the red dye #40 that is still in use is a coal-tar derivative as well. It's already been banned in other countries of the world. Coal-tar derivatives are proved carcinogens. In his book, *The Greatest Battle,* Dr. Ronald Glasser reveals the startling fact that a 110-pound woman could absorb enough of such a coal-tar derivative to reach dangerous blood levels by drinking as little as a third of a can of grape soda daily, and that a child could exceed the recognized safe limit with just a couple of gulps from the same can of pop.

All things considered, soda is definitely *not* a good way to quench your thirst!

COFFEE, TEA, AND CHOCOLATE CONTAIN STIMULANTS THAT LOWER YOUR VITALITY AND HEALTH LEVEL. Coffee, tea, and chocolate all contain a substance called *theobromine.* It's an irritant, or stimulant, and has an affinity especially for your brain cells. Remember, anything that artificially stimulates causes extra stress! Such stress leads to premature aging and breakdown of your faithful cells.

FIVE REASONS WHY COFFEE ISN'T GOOD FOR YOU.

1) It contains caffeine, a drug that has been found to inhibit activity of the enzyme DNA polymerase, the code material of your cells. Ultimately caffeine can interfere with your memory, because it harms this coding part of your cells, which sends out messages.

2) Coffee has a pyridine base. The breakdown product of this

chemical in your body is urea, the same toxic residue you get when you eat meat. Charles Eliot Perkins, a biochemist who's done extensive research in cancer, has found that the one substance that's common to all cancer-producing chemical compounds and without which there can be no cancer activity, is pyridine. It's the same chemical that's found in coal-tar, soot, and tobacco smoke.

3) Excessive coffee drinking can cause your heart to race (tachycardia) and, if you're high-strung or under emotional stress, can cause cardiac pain.

4) It has a diuretic effect on your kidneys, as they speed up their work of filtering out as best they can the harmful chemicals it contains.

5) It's addicting. Coffee causes constriction of the blood vessels in your brain. It's this sort of constriction that can lead to high blood pressure. When you miss your regular coffee time, you'll get a headache as your blood vessels begin to dilate. Coffee drinkers often get headaches the first day of a fast due to withdrawal of their drug.

WHAT ABOUT TEA AND CHOCOLATE?

Tea contains a substance called theine which is very similar to caffeine. It contains, in addition, a substance called *tannic acid* which has a diuretic effect, causing your kidneys to overwork. The theine in tea also causes dispepsia, or indigestion.

The theobromine in chocolate is a poisonous alkaloid—the same drug that's found in morphine, cocaine, quinine, and strychnine. In sensitive people theobromine can trigger skin rashes, sinus attacks, headaches, and asthma attacks.

Coffee, tea, and chocolate drinks are not a healthy way to quench your thirst.

MILK IS A PERFECT FOOD—FOR BABIES!

Humans are the only animals that drink milk throughout their lives. The young of each species are provided with nourishment which is perfectly suited to their own special needs. As civilization progresses and mothers become more sophisticated and less healthy, they have given over their jobs more and more to cows. Children, consequently, have grown larger and developed sooner than old-fashioned mother's milk-fed babies. In addition, they've never been weaned. Animals in nature nurse only until they have enough teeth to chew their own food. It seems logical that human babies should, too, does it not?

Cow's milk contains more protein, more sugar, salt, and fat, and less water than mother's milk. It was designed to sustain a larger animal. Our children have responded to a high intake of this food by growing larger. This is, in reality, forced growth, with a consequent lowering of the quality of health.

After the age of about four, the production of renin in the child's body is stopped. (Renin is the secretion manufactured in the thymus gland which is responsible for the coagulation of milk.) About this same age, the intestinal enzyme lactase, which is responsible for the digestion of the milk sugar lactose, disappears from humans' digestive tracts.

These changes coincide roughly with the age at which a child can chew its own food and be well nourished without milk. From then on, the child can make its own calcium from green plants, fruits, and vegetables, as other young primates can. Evidence points to the fact that milk drinking beyond this stage, all things being equal, can cause problems.

» Overconsumption of milk is one of the causes of childhood obesity.
» Brings on the early onset of atherosclerosis—sludge in the arteries—a condition which contributes to the high incidence of heart disease in both men and women at younger and younger ages.
» Causes diarrhea, indigestion, infections, and certain allergies.

Stop the milk drinking and get your calcium and amino acids first hand, as my family and I have done for over thirty years. It will save on your milk *and* doctor bills!

ALCOHOL IS A DEPRESSANT DRUG.

A martini before lunch gets you in a friendly mood. You can even *enjoy* clinching a deal with a recalcitrant client.

A couple of scotches on ice with a whisper of water, and the bores around you at a cocktail party become beautiful. A few glasses of vintage wine throughout your meal enables you to forget your shyness and you become a sparkling conversationalist. You also eat twice as much as you intended to.

If you're the kind of person who can do this occasionally and not make it a habit—a habit that may eventually lead from one to three martinis with lunch, or an entire bottle of wine at a sitting—

you're lucky. Even if you are lucky enough to avoid addiction you should know what alcohol consumption does to your body.

Ten reasons why you should avoid alcohol.

1) *Alcohol impairs the proper functioning of your entire metabolic process.* Yet, ironically, studies show that the particular type of malnutrition produced by the high-calorie, concentrated, unnatural diet prevalent in America today predisposes you toward drinking alcohol. A diet high in processed food content creates an imbalance of vitamins and minerals. Your cells are more likely to "yell out" for the artificial stimulation of alcohol, substituting for the missing elements they really need. This creates more deficiencies and metabolic malfunctioning in your system. It perpetuates the cycle.

2) Evidence points strongly to the possibility that *alcohol weakens your heart muscle.* This condition is called "cardiomyopathy." In experiments on rats, even those on healthy diets developed fatty, enlarged hearts when they were given regular amounts of alcohol.

3) *Alcohol causes intoxication of your brain cells.* When taken in any quantity it damages both individual brain cells and groups of brain cells. The first part of your brain to be affected is the outer layer, which controls worry and anxiety. Higher alcohol levels affect the motor area of your brain which controls your muscular systems. Even higher levels affect your mid-brain and may cause you to go into a stupor. The ultimate damage could be death.

4) *Alcohol causes the red cells in your blood to clump together.* The outer thin covering of each of your cells serves to protect them and to give them shape. It also sends out electrical charges which in effect is a signaling system, controlling the arrangement of the cells. Alcohol interferes with this cellular membrane. It causes the rearrangement of the electrical charges of your red blood cells' cellular membranes. The cells change shape. The plus and minus charges don't work right and the cells become attracted to each other and begin to clump together. When these clumps reach your blood vessels or capillaries, the vessels, especially the smaller ones, get clogged, preventing vital oxygen from getting through. Hemorrhaging is frequently the result.

This is what's happening when your eyes become bloodshot.

This is what's happening in chronic alcoholics whose noses turn red.

This is what's happening in your brain cells when you get a

headache after drinking. Oxygen is being denied these vital cells. They *die* when this happens. They can never be replaced. The brain of the chronic drinker becomes permanently impaired.

5) *Chronic drinking depresses sexual functioning.* While alcohol in small amounts loosens you up and puts you in a more relaxed (literally more depressed) state, freeing your emotional response, extensive studies prove conclusively that it depresses sexual performance. If you have a long history of drinking alcohol, evidence is in which shows you'll tend toward premature senility. This means premature impotency and degeneration of your sexual organs.

6) *Alcohol injures cellular membranes.* This makes them more vulnerable to the effects of other potentially harmful chemicals that may be floating around in your extra-cellular fluid. Once inside the nucleus of your cells, some chemicals jam up the works, interfering with the coding system which maintains law and order. This can trigger a state of anarchy among cells, which is what the cancer process is all about. Once triggered, this process is irreversible.

7) *If you drink, statistics show you're much more likely to smoke.* This places you in double jeopardy.

8) *Liver damage is prevalent among steady drinkers.* Your liver is the hardest working, most indispensable organ in your body next to your heart. Alcohol interferes with its healthy functioning.

9) Studies show that pregnant women who drink are prone to give birth to babies with serious birth defects. Men, don't sit back and relax thinking it's only what your wife or lover does that will affect the quality of your offspring. Recent experiments lead to the conclusion that *heavy-drinking fathers produce alcohol-damaged sperm.* Your drinking may cause your mate to abort, or to give birth to a defective child.

10) *The capacity to think clearly is interfered with* when you drink, affecting your efficiency and impairing your ability to concentrate.

Summing it up, we can say, then, that alcoholic beverages are the kind of thirst quenchers that can also be life-quenchers!

FRUIT JUICES ARE A FOOD AND SHOULDN'T BE TAKEN INDISCRIMINATELY.

As a rule it's best to eat fruits and vegetables whole. Fruits and vegetables are surrounded with a tough outer capsule or skin that's designed as an effective barrier against oxidation. When this is broken, they begin to oxidize and to loose some of their food value. Oranges, for instance, loose important amounts of vitamin C once they're cut and juiced. When you do juice them, it's best to drink the juice right away, as the longer it's kept the more oxidation takes place. Frozen concentrates, aside from loosing vitamin C through oxidation, have had benzoic acid and sodium benzoate added as preservatives. Sulphur dioxide is another toxic chemical that's used as a preservative in these concentrates.

There are times when juices are both thirst quenching and satisfying. They contain essential vitamins and minerals and provide these while at the same time providing your system with the fluid it needs for proper water balance. Once in awhile, after exertion when I feel the need for a fast pick-up, I'll have a glass of fresh juice. I make it a practice to have it alone. Fruit juice is an excellent alternative to soft drinks, candy bars, and other refined carbohydrates as an instant energizer.

When you eat a predominance of fresh raw juicy fruits, succulent vegetables, no salt and spices and little or no meat, you'll find you rarely get thirsty. Succulent fruits and vegetables will provide your system with all the highly vitaminized, mineralized water it needs. This nutritious water will be used in your bloodstream and by your cells not only to provide the correct water balance necessary for optimal body functioning, but in addition will supply the fiber and bulk needed for prevention of bowel problems and constipation. Mother nature has thought of everything in the packaging of tender, juicy, nutritious food for you. It's when you interfere with her judicious planning and packaging and take your food apart and cook, process, preserve, and add sugar, salt, and chemicals to it that you get in trouble.

WHEN YOU LOSE WATER FROM YOUR SYSTEM FROM SWEATING, DRINKING PURE WATER IS THE BEST WAY TO RESTORE THE LOST WATER.

Physical exertion such as jogging, running, or working in the hot sun are instances when unusual thirst calls for water drinking. If you feel, after having had water, that it's insufficient, pure fresh orange juice or a piece of watermelon will bring your water *and* sugar levels back to par.

DRINKING SEVERAL GLASSES OF WATER A DAY DOES NOT FLUSH TOXINS OUT OF YOUR SYSTEM. It's a myth that drinking large amounts of water will flush toxins out of your system. Excess water drinking raises the volume of fluid in your bloodstream. This causes

» higher blood pressure (headaches)
» more work for your kidneys
» dilution of the minerals in your bloodstream, thus reducing their effectiveness.

CHAPTER 10

How to Make Your New Diet a Way of Life

Children and the New Eating Plan

Introducing children to the Born-Again regime will take patience and persistence. It's important to sit down with them and discuss the new plan, share your inspiration and motivation with them, and point out how eating differently from their friends will have advantages. It will help them to avoid being sick, overweight, and troubled with skin problems.

Here are some things you can do to help your children make the switch to new, healthy food habits more easily.

» Have regular family discussions about the new eating plan and how everyone's reacting to it. Encourage them to express themselves openly.

» Keep fresh fruit, dried fruit, raw nuts, unprocessed cheeses, and natural fruit juices on hand at all times.

» Use the blender to make fresh fruit shakes.

» Allow concessions when they have their friends over—wholewheat pasta, frozen fruit yogurt, zucchini bread, or whatever they like that's not made from refined foods. (Kids will usually realize sooner or later that their friends are perfectly happy with fresh fruit and nuts and other natural goodies that they can't get at *their* houses.)

» Take the children on health convention vacations where vegetarians and other health-minded families go. It helps when they meet other young people who're involved in healthful living. The American Natural Hygiene Society, 1920 Irving Park Road, Chicago, Illinois 60613, has such a convention every year. They are pleasant, informative occasions usually held on college campuses. You live in dorms and are served natural vegetarian meals cafeteria style.

» Try a health resort with your youngsters if you can afford it. I spent last Thanksgiving at the Shangri-La in Bonita Springs, Florida, with my seventeen-year-old daughter. She prodded *me* to go!

» Be sure to let your teenagers know how much confidence you have in them. Instead of nagging, praise each good choice they make. Don't panic if you find out that they're experimenting with drugs or alcohol. Encourage them to talk with you about it.

» Stress good foods, but not to the exclusion of other important elements of healthy living. Encourage participation in gymnastics, acrobatics, dance, sports.

HOW TO INFLUENCE WHAT YOUR CHILDREN GET TO EAT AT CAMPS AND PRIVATE SCHOOLS. Louis, my oldest child, attended private boarding school most of his school years. His early nutritional training must have stood him in good stead, for he refused all flesh foods throughout those years. We had an understanding with the school that he be allowed to indulge in as much salad and fresh fruit as they could provide. In between times we sent along care packages of dried fruits, nuts, and other natural snacks.

When David went to camp in the summer I left extra weekly money with the camp director for the purchase of fresh fruit and vegetables for David. This arrangement worked fine.

Whenever my children have gone away to camp I've managed to get assurances from the camps that the children will have a selection of vegetarian foods at mealtimes—salads, potatoes, and whole grain bread. You can do the same for your children. When enough parents and kids let camp directors know their preferences, changes away from the starchy foodplans will begin to be made.

NATURAL FOOD AT PARTIES. Children love parties. They're special and they're fun. You can make a party special without resorting to ice cream and chocolate cake.

Slice a big round section from the center of a ripe red juicy watermelon, putting candles on it as if it were a cake.

Make an uncooked fruit cake and decorate it with candles. Here's the recipe:

1 pound pitted dates
½ pound currants
¾ cup of lightly roasted almonds
1 carrot

Put ingredients through a food grinder and then mix together 2 tablespoons of sesame seeds, 2 tablespoons of freshly grated coconut, and, if desired, 1 tablespoon carob powder. Shape the dried fruit mix into a square on a cake plate and cover with the seed mixture, patting onto top and sides. Decorate with whole almonds or pecans. (Courtesy Fay Morris, Toronto, Canada.)

If your child wants a more conventional birthday cake, make a carrot or banana cake, using whole-wheat flower and brown sugar instead of the white flower and sugar called for in the recipe.

How to Help Your Mate Switch Over to the New Diet

Here are some simple ways to begin getting your mate to appreciate the new way of eating.

1) Broil foods instead of frying.

2) Reduce the number of times a week you serve meat.

3) Tempt him or her with interesting salads.

4) Get some good vegetarian cookbooks and begin learning how to prepare interesting vegetarian dishes.

5) Make mealtime pleasant and serve your new fruit and vegetable dishes as attractively as possible.

6) Most important of all, be a good example. Remember you have every right to eat the way you think is best for *you*. NEVER eat to please anyone but yourself. Don't allow anyone else to make you feel guilty.

Eating Out

So many people say to me, "How could I ever stick to a vegetarian regime? I like eating out too much."

Eating out and eating right are not really difficult at all. Most good restaurants have wonderful salads these days. Ask for the Caesar salad without dressing and then dress it yourself with oil and lemon. Or order a chef's salad and ask them to leave off the meat and cheese. Or ask for a triple-sized mixed green salad.

A restaurant in our area has a great salad bar except that they use white head lettuce, which hasn't much in the way of nutrients. I carry a plastic bag of watercress, or romaine, or both, as well as a sandwich bag of sprouts with me when we go there for dinner. When no one's noticing I reinforce my salad bowl with my own goodies. I've been known to take along my own vegetable powder and lemon and add it to their oil. Lately this restaurant has begun to serve greener, more nutritious lettuce. Who knows? Perhaps Ed, the owner, caught me reinforcing my salad!

Eating at Friends' Homes

You may be nervous about letting your friends know you've decided to change your eating habits, and that you won't be eating the roast beef or chicken or fancy desserts when you have dinner in their homes. Don't be nervous. Your friends will understand. Ours have learned over the years that we're quite happy to make our meal off the trimmings—salad, vegetables, cheese, or potato. Now they make larger salads when they know we're coming. They put out fresh fruit along with the dessert.

At cocktail parties you can carry a glass of orange juice around. Or you can order a virgin mary (tomato juice with a twist of lemon) or a presbyterian (club soda with an olive). If you want to deviate a bit, nurse a glass of white wine.

Entertaining Your Friends

Changing your eating habits doesn't mean you have to put a stop to your entertaining. I've done a great deal of party-giving over the years and have learned to prepare wonderful, festive meals for others who may not share my lifestyle. Here are a few of my party menus:

LUNCHEON #1

Waldorf Salad
Cheese soufflé
Steamed baby peas
Fresh fruit, nuts

DINNER #1

Huge tossed green salad
Spanish Casserole
Steamed whole green beans
Yellow squash à la Joy
Raspberry yogurt (optional)

LUNCHEON #2

Tossed green salad
Crepes Florentine
Steamed fresh asparagus
Fresh fruit compote

DINNER #2

Spinach and mushroom salad
Stuffed zucchini
Green baby limas
Steamed broccoli
Berry Bowl with whipped cream

LUNCHEON #3	*DINNER #3*
Cream of zucchini soup	Joy's celery soup
Stuffed celery	Creamy baked corn
Tomato salad	Large green salad
Sliced strawberries with whipped cream	Steamed Brussels sprouts
	Fresh fruit

CHAPTER 11

How to Pick Perfect Fruits and Vegetables

FRESH FRUITS AND VEGETABLES ARE THE DELECTABLE MAIN-STAY OF YOUR NEW LIFETIME EATING PLAN. Just glance at the Month of Menus at the end of this section and you'll get the idea immediately. From now on in your life it's going to be fruits and vegetables galore! I'll teach you new ways of cooking them, new ways of arranging them raw so you won't have to bother cooking them at all. With what you learn in this section you'll be able to expand, infinitely, your repertoire of good, wholesome, "live" foods. You'll try out vegetables you've never had before, order exotic fruits by mail. You'll learn to make tantalizing salads you can eat as much as you want of and still lose pounds. I'll share with you my favorite, ten-minute, vegetable soup recipes. There is a whole new world of gustatory delights waiting for you out there, and it bears no resemblance at all to your childhood recollection of mother saying, "Eat your vegetables!" as she served up yet another helping of blackened, soupy, overcooked spinach.

SOON YOU'LL BE SAVORING VEGETABLES AND FRUITS THE WAY OTHERS SAVOR MEATS AND DESSERTS. I tell you, I've been eating this way for years and its appeal has never diminished. I still can't get over the fantastic array of colors, textures, and tastes my garden produces for me each summer: cauliflower, with its nutlike crunch, the rich, heavy flesh of tomatoes in season, tiny niblets of sweet corn straight from the cob, deep green broccoli so tender you can happily forget cooking it. And as for desserts, nothing beats nature's bounty of fruits, melons, and berries. It's as rich and varied as the pastry tray in any fancy French restaurant.

On the other hand, I can understand how someone might be less than enthusiastic about a diet made up largely of fruits and vegetables, unless what you were getting was simply the best available—what I call "prime." As meat lovers look for prime cuts, so, too, do vegetable lovers want top quality. "Prime" produce is perfect produce—sweet, succulent, fine-flavored. Anything less (slightly mushy, not fully sweet, on the tasteless side) is not worth your time or money.

And speaking of money! Don't do yourself the disservice of trying to scrimp on your food budget. Remember, you're going to cut out—entirely, or at least largely—the most expensive items you used to buy: meat, poultry, and fish. So pamper yourself. Eat raspberries out of season whenever you can get your hands on them. Order juicy citrus fruits by the case directly from Florida (or through your local Agway store, if you live rurally.) If tropical fruits—mangoes and papaya—aren't available where you live, order them from Florida, too. (See appendix B) The point is this: no matter how extravagant a lover of fruits and vegetables you become, your food budget will *never* exceed the meat eater's. So go out, find the best, and load up your refrigerator. Indulge!

WHERE TO FIND "PRIME" FRUITS AND VEGETABLES. If you live in the country, as I do, you can grow your own. Or, if you haven't the time or the inclination to garden, you can find wonderful produce at local farm stands.

While supermarket produce in general tends not to be superior, you can still do well by striking up a good business relationship with the produce buyer at your supermarket. He may be able to order things especially for you—persimmons, fresh figs. Or, because he does a big volume business, he may be willing to alter his prices for you in order to meet the price of a competitor. When I found Hawaiian pineapples for sale cheaper at another market, I told my regular supermarket produce man and he promptly made the very same brand of pineapples available to me at the competitor's lower price. I almost always buy my fruits and vegetables in quantity, however. It's doubtful that Bernie, my produce man, would have lowered his price had I only wanted a single pineapple.

I bought a case of twelve and we had fresh pineapple juice for a week.

If you live in the city, there's probably a big outdoor market somewhere. It's worth it to go there and take a cab home with a week's worth of produce if you can't find the good stuff close by. Probably, though, you can. Most city neighborhoods have at least one shop or sidewalk stand that specializes in prime fruits and vegetables. Usually these places are supplied by farms in outlying rural areas. The farmers truck their produce in, fresh from the fields, every morning.

Now, what to look for when selecting your prime produce. Nothing is more disappointing than to whack into a big, expensive honeydew, only to find that it's not *quite* ripe, it's just a *bit* on the hard side, its flavor is just a *trifle* underdeveloped. (In some ways it's less frustrating if the melon's completely green.) Nothing is more annoying than to buy fresh corn and discover, when you bite into it, that it's tough and starchy . . . or to buy green beans that look decent enough in the store but go limp and withered the instant you get them home. Regardless of where you end up doing your shopping, there are certain unmistakable signs of prime quality. I'm going to describe them for you here. Look for them when selecting your fruits and vegetables.

Vegetables

Asparagus should be on the slender side, and deep green with a nice, tight head. The shaft should be smooth and unridged, and not in the least limp or dusty-colored. Before cooking (or eating raw), break the fibrous end of the shaft off where it snaps naturally. What you have left (the longer portion of the shaft) is prime.

Beans and fresh peas should be so crisp they give a good "crack" when you snap them in two. If they seem at all flexible, pass them by.

The cabbage family includes broccoli, Brussels sprouts, and cauliflower, as well as cabbage. (Tests on laboratory animals indicate a diet high in these cruciferous vegetables may reduce the risk of cancer.) Both cauliflower and broccoli are the buds of the plants, basically, and should be tightly closed, not on the verge of flowering. Cauliflower should have no brown spots and broccoli no yellow.

Brussels sprouts should be bright green with no faded, loose edges on the leaves. While the main head of the cabbage should be tight and solid, its outer leaves can be loose, as long as they seem crisp and vigorous.

Carrots stay fresh a long time. So do their cousins, parsnips and turnips. As long as these vegetables are good and solid with fresh, bright color, they're usually fine.

Corn starts converting its natural sugar to starch the minute it's picked, so go for the absolute freshest you can find. The signs are clear. The outer leaves should be green and tightly folded; the silk should be brown and dry, without a trace of sliminess. When you pull down the leaves a bit from the top, to check the condition of the kernels, you should find them uniform in size and color, with no dents in the center to signify overripeness. Press a kernel with your thumbnail. If it spurts, the corn is fresh and sweet.

Cucumbers are often waxed so they'll hold their moisture longer. Try to avoid them (they smear when you rub them) because un-waxed cucumbers can be eaten peel and all and are much more nutritious. The small, pickle cukes two or three inches long are the best.

Green peppers should be firm, dark green, and without soft or brown spots. Check the stem end, which withers first.

Lettuce heads should feel firm and solid, for the most part. Boston and Bibb lettuce have softer, more delicate leaves than romaine or iceberg, but the leaves should show no signs of wilt. Romaine is the darkest green, with long leaves and high in vitamins and amino acids. It should have no rust spots near the top edges. The loose, leaf lettuce from spring and summer gardens is also high in nutritional value. Its leaves will be tender but should not be wilted.

Onions should be hard and firm. Don't buy them if their smell is very strong. It means they're going to sprout soon.

Parsley should be bright green and crisp. I prefer buying it in bunches rather than mashed down under plastic wrap in a package.

Potatoes should have clear, unblemished skins and should feel quite hard, without any signs of sprouts.

Spinach should be bought the way it grows, in clumps—not in cellophane bags, if possible. Its leaves should be large, dark green, and crisp.

Summer squash has tender skin and doesn't keep fresh very long. Green zucchini, yellow crookneck or straight-neck should be brightly colored. When small and slender they're firm and crisp and have smaller seeds and more flavor.

Sweet potatoes and yams should have bright, clear skins. They don't keep long and shouldn't be refrigerated because it turns them limp.

Tomatoes are always best when in season and home or farm-grown. Beefsteak tomatoes should be nice and red and on the firm side (never mushy). If you live in an area where you can't get home-growns in winter, choose the firm, red hothouse varieties over those sickly hydroponics that come prepackaged. Hothouse tomatoes are more expensive, but they're worth it.

Winter squash—acorn, butternut, and Hubbard—keep a long time at room temperature and longer, refrigerated, because they have hard, tough rinds. Don't buy them unless their stems are firmly attached, however, for a winter squash without its stem is on the way out.

Watercress is delicate and won't last long. It should have shiny, deep green leaves and look quite sprightly. Watercress that's limp when you buy it is going to be stringy and harsh tasting.

Perfect Fruit

Serving perfectly ripened fruits and melons can mean the difference between success and failure in your new Eating Plan. They should be sweet, succulent, and totally satisfying.

Avocados (yes, they're a fruit!) should be firm, never mushy. The pear-shaped California variety is a more concentrated fruit and has a thinner skin. It should be firm but not hard to the touch, yielding to a bit of gentle probing. The rounder, Florida variety has a tougher skin and is a bit more watery in texture. Select it as you would the pear-shaped variety.

Bananas can be bought when they're light yellow and stored in a dark cupboard until they become speckled lightly with brown. Speckling indicates they've changed from starch to sugar (just the opposite of what corn does once it's picked). At this stage they're digested more easily. In selecting prime bananas, watch out for bruises and soft spots on otherwise firm fruit.

Citrus fruits—grapefruit, oranges, tangerines—should feel heavy for their size (a sign of juice). Oranges kept in cold storage are available throughout the year but their true season begins in early November. A greenish cast in an orange is a good sign because it means the fruit hasn't been dyed. Grapefruit are sometimes sun-freckled, a sign of extra sweetness. Tangerines are prime when they feel just a bit loose in their skins but not pulpy around the ends.

Fresh figs are in season July, August, and September. Both purple and white figs should be plump and soft to the touch. The softer they are without actually being rotten or moldy, the sweeter they'll be.

Grapes vary according to type. Tokays (my favorite) have a lamentably short season. My market carries them for only three or four weeks at the end of October. They should be quite firm, and of a robust, orchid color. Emperors look quite a bit like Tokays but tend to be smaller, less firm, and available for a longer season. Ribiers are large, blue-black grapes that are exquisitely flavorful, though their seeds are large. Buy them when they're still firm. The Thompson seedless is a small, white grape. It should be firm and yellowish in color. When its color is more green than yellow it's not yet fully ripe.

Mangoes, in my opinion, are nature's juiciest, most heavenly treat. The ones more commonly shipped to northern markets are the Hayden variety, a large, oval-shaped fruit. It is ripe when it's heavily yellow and orange-streaked, firm, yet yielding to gentle thumb pressure. The Carrie is a green variety. When ripe, it simply turns a paler green and begins to develop dark, brownish-black speckles at the stem end. It, too, should be firm, yet yield to pressure.

Melons (honeydew, casaba, Spanish, Persian, and Crenshaw) are ripe when the flat end opposite the stem end yields easily to gentle thumb pressure. If there's only a hint of its giving to pressure, buy the melon and store it in the pantry (not refrigerator) for several days until the end becomes softer.

Cantaloupe should be yellow all over and smell deliciously aromatic, yet still be firm to the touch. Cantaloupes that are greenish and hard are almost invariably inedible.

Watermelon should pass the thump test. When you plunk it with your thumb and forefinger you should get a mellow, full-sounding thump that tells you it's at its prime.

Papayas should be firm yet give to the touch. Buy them either yellow-streaked or all yellow. If they're dark green and hard in the market, it means they were so green when they were picked that they'll start to rot before they ripen.

Nectarines should be picked for firmness (not hardness) and for color. The more red-streaked, usually, the sweeter.

Peaches, plums, pears are, like nectarines, tree fruits. They're best when local and tree-ripened. If you purchase them slightly under-ripe, you'll avoid dents from other people's fingers. These fruits can do their final ripening in your home. Pears should have a slightly greenish cast. Peaches should not. Plums should have no brownish patches.

Pineapples are best when they're from Hawaii. The Puerto Rican and Honduran varieties simply aren't as sweet, and tend to be tasteless and woody in texture. The Hawaiian variety is sugar-sweet, juicy, and delicious. A pineapple should be firm, with a yellowish glow under the skin, and no dark spots. You should be able to pluck a top leaf easily from its moorings. You should also be able to get the aroma of pineapple when you sniff its bottom end.

Storage Tips

Don't wash more *lettuce* than you can use in two days for it will begin to "bleed" at the bottom of its center rib and turn rusty. This means that oxidation is taking place and vitamins are getting lost.

It's far more conducive to lettuce and salad-eating to have your lettuce prepared ahead of time—cleaned, dried, crisped. When I get home from the market I fill my sink halfway with cold water, cut the base off the Romaine, discard spotted or yellowish outer leaves, separate the rest and immerse them in the cold water. If you swish the leaves around gently you'll get rid of dirt and sand. Let the water out of the sink, fill it up a second time, and repeat the process. (Boston and leaf lettuce may require additional washings, as they usually trap more sand and dirt in their bottom leaves. The same is true of spinach. Change waters until the bottom of the sink is absolutely grit-free.)

After the lettuce has been washed, shake it out gently and arrange the leaves on a terry towel. Take another terry towel and pat the leaves. I roll the lettuce in the towel and shake it gently over the sink. When the lettuce leaves are good and dry I transfer them to large plastic bags and secure at the top with twisters. Lettuce stored this way will keep crisp and fresh for several days.

Parsley, watercress, and *broccoli* stay green and fresh longer if you stand them up in a container of cold water in the refrigerator.

Parsley and watercress are sometimes sandy and should be held under a trickle of water from the faucet until clean, then dried before storing.

Fruit is something I don't wash until just before it's to be eaten. Washing fruit and berries before storing tends to cause it to decompose sooner. If you select your fruits carefully (using the guidelines above) and then store them in a dry, dark place like the pantry, they'll ripen as you use them, day by day. Refrigerated fruits lose the fullness of flavor that room-temperature fruits have so don't refrigerate unless you're afraid the fruit is going to spoil.

Never refrigerate bananas. I have a trick for bananas that are on the verge of overripeness. I make up banana bread and freeze it for guests' use *or* I cut each ripe banana in three sections, store in a plastic bag, and freeze the sections until such time as I want to drop them in a blender, along with some juice, for a fruitshake.

Dried fruit, nuts, and *seeds* are less likely to have been fumigated against bug infestation or to have had preservatives added when you buy them from your local health food store or food co-op. If you buy them in any quantity you can keep them fresh by storing nuts and seeds in your freezer and dried fruits in your refrigerator.

Cooking for the Born-Again Body

In general, cooking tends to destroy the vitamins and minerals in foods. It can also change protein molecules, making them tougher and harder to be absorbed through your cell walls and into your cells. Some foods, however (like potatoes and grains) need to be lightly cooked because our enzymes can't break them down sufficiently for digestion. There's a method of cooking that drastically reduces the loss of nutrients. It calls for special cookware.

BUYING QUALITY COOKWARE IS AN INVESTMENT IN YOUR OWN FUTURE. What you need are utensils that spread heat quickly and evenly and also hold heat, and that have covers that seal tightly without being locked on. These qualities allow for minimal oxidation and you can cook vegetables until they're tender with very little or no water, and low, low temperatures, and in the shortest possible period of time. This way you retain flavor and lose as few vitamins and minerals as possible.

The best cookware is a kind of stainless steel alloy called No. 304 stainless steel. It's noncontaminating and is widely used in the food-processing and wine-making industries. Vessels made with it will be stamped as such. They are constructed with inner layers of carbon steel on the sides and bottoms of pans, and inner layers of aluminum sandwiched in the bottom as well. (The very best cookware will have no carbon steel or aluminum visible to the eye.)

Not long ago, the Home Economics Department of the Buffalo *Courier Express* did a study of nutrient-retaining cooking methods. The newspaper gave tips on buying cookware. "Quality in cookware is measured by the number of layers it has," the paper noted. "The more layers, the better the quality. Try to get over five plies (layers)."

With many-layered stainless steel cookware you can use very little or no water at all. The theory behind this kind of cooking is that heat is stored in the walls and bottoms of the vessels as uniformly as possible. You can start the vegetable dry, over medium heat, and it will soon begin to "sweat." This moisture will form a vapor seal between the edge of the pot and a properly weighted and balanced cover. At this point the temperature from the burner is reduced, creating a semi-vacuum inside the pot. When cooked in a semi-vacuum, vegetables can be tenderized at considerably lower temperatures (between 170° and 180° F.) than under other conditions. In short, you can tenderize vegetables without even boiling them!

Unfortunately, first rate cookware that can be used in this way is not available everywhere. There *is* some you can send away for, however. It's called Lifetime (write for their catalogue) and it's six-ply stainless steel cookware. The addrss is P.O. Box 5693, San Jose, California 95150.

If you're not prepared to replace all your cookware (it can be quite an investment, though a worthwhile one) here's how I steam vegetables with my own cookware, which is tightly lidded and stainless. You'll need a steaming basket or trivet to place inside your pots for steaming. A quarter- to a half-cup of water is necessary with this method, depending upon the quantity of vegetable you're cooking. (Two cups of fresh string beans would require ½ cup of water; 1 cup of beans would need only ¼ cup.) Place string beans, or any other cut up vegetable, inside a steaming basket (this keeps the vegetable from touching the water) inside an uncovered pot. Quickly bring the water to a boil, reduce the heat to low, and put on a tight lid. After 5 minutes, turn the heat off and allow the beans to remain in the pan with the lid on for a few more minutes, until tender. Serve at once.

Grain foods such as kasha, or buckwheat groats, require more water and more time. Using a ratio of 3 parts water to 1 grain, drop kasha or groats into boiling water, put on the tight lid, and turn off the heat. Within ten or fifteen minutes the grain will be tender and fluffy.

Other grain foods take varying amounts of time. All the grain recipes included in this book are accompanied by steaming instructions.

CHAPTER 12

Ten Salads You Can Eat All You Want of and Still Lose Weight

For most of us, dieting to lose weight is a real challenge to the will. Even when you've reached your ideal weight and are simply trying to hold the battle line, there are times when you get the urge to sit down and eat to your heart's content, without counting calories, without worrying about protein content, or vitamins, or minerals. What you want is to be able to eat, guilt-free, until you're completely satisfied.

The good news is that there's a way to do this. It's salad! Not only are salad greens low in calories (a big leaf of romaine has only 2 calories), they're rich in vitamins, minerals, and that super energizer, chlorophyl. Greens also contain all the essential amino acids but one, and that one (methionine) you can get, as noted, by eating small quantities of seeds a few times a week.

AS LONG AS YOU KNOW HOW TO MAKE IT THE NATURAL WAY, YOU CAN EAT AS MUCH SALAD AS YOU LIKE. No mayonnaise or other goopy dressings, please. No hunks of cheese, or croutons, or bits of bacon, whether synthetic or real. Train your taste buds to enjoy the simple flavors of greens as nature grew them. Learn to make what I call "natural" dressings. As you'll see, all of my dressing recipes use cold pressed, unsaturated oils. (Hain and Erewhon are good brands. Most health food stores and some supermarkets carry them.) The refined, chemically treated oils usually found on your supermarket shelf won't do. They're high in saturated fats and processed for a long shelf life, not a long human life.

Use lemon juice instead of vinegar. Vinegar irritates your digestive tract and inhibits the normal flow of gastric juices, which hampers digestion.

Begin training your taste buds to appreciate the flavor of salads without salt. As you probably know, salt makes you retain fluids and is poison to your system. If you must have seasoning, I recommend a vegetable powder, Vegebase, or Sherman's Arcadia soup base, all of which can be gotten in health food stores.

All right. Gather your ingredients together, get out your salad bowl, and get ready to dig in. The ten wonderful salad recipes that follow may look extremely simple—and they are! But you'll find them delicious and satisfying. Eat as much as you like and grow healthier with each biteful.

BASIC BORN-AGAIN SALAD
1 medium-size head of romaine lettuce

Start with washed, crisp lettuce. Break the leaves into bite-size pieces, toss with basic dressing and garnish, if you like, with ripe tomato wedges, cucumber slices, and rings of thinly sliced spanish onion. Sprinkle with a little dill, freshly chopped or dried. This salad serves one very adequately.

MIXED GREEN SALAD
½ a head of romaine
1 small head of Boston lettuce
Several leaves of curly endive
A few sprigs of parsley
1 cup of alfalfa sprouts

Break the different lettuces into bite-size pieces. Add parsley and sprouts and toss with basic dressing.

MIXED VEGETABLE SALAD
1 medium head of romaine
¼ of a large or ½ of a small green or red ripe pepper
1 stalk celery
4 or 5 plum tomatoes
½ a cucumber, thinly sliced
1 scallion
1 carrot, grated

Break romaine into bite-size pieces. Add slivered green pepper, celery, tomatoes, cucumber, and scallion (including the good green top). Dress with vege-dressing and top with grated carrot.

SPINACH SALAD
1 quart of carefully washed and dried spinach leaves
1 cup of thinly-sliced raw mushrooms
½ cup alfalfa sprouts
4 ripe olives

If spinach leaves are large, tear them into bite-size pieces; otherwise, leave them whole. Add mushrooms, toss with basic dressing, and garnish with sprouts and olives.

RAINBOW SALAD
1 medium head of romaine
2 raw asparagus spears
1 cup of thinly sliced red cabbage
½ carrot, thinly sliced
½ a small, tender raw yellow squash
1 scallion

Break romaine into bite-size pieces in salad bowl. Add slivered vegetables. Toss lightly with either cottage cheese or basic dressing.

FINGER SALAD
2 spears fresh broccoli
20 whole fresh green beans
12 leaves romaine lettuce
3 or 4 whole leaves of Boston lettuce
2 stalks celery
4 carrot sticks
1 ripe tomato

Steam the broccoli spears and whole green beans until just tender. (Follow instructions in how-to-steam section.) They should be tender but hard, and quite green. Cool. Arrange ingredients so they are standing up in a tall bowl and serve with avocado dressing on the side, which you can use as a dip. This large, filling salad including ½ cup of dressing, contains 236 calories—less than 3 ounces of roast beef!

SUPER SPROUTS
12 large crisped spinach leaves
16 ounces alfalfa sprouts
6 ripe plum tomatoes or one large tomato cut in wedges

Arrange spinach leaves around salad bowl with tops overlapping outside edge of the bowl. Fill the bowl with sprouts and arrange tomato at the bottom of the bowl between the spinach leaves and the sprouts. Pour your favorite natural dressing over the sprouts and crunch away.

WATERCRESS SPECIAL
1 large bunch crisp clean watercress
1 small head Boston lettuce
¼ cup chopped parsley
½ cup sliced fresh mushrooms

Toss lightly with 1½ tbsp. safflower oil, 1 tbsp. Vegebase, and the juice of ¼ a lemon. If you can find fresh arugula in your area, you may substitute that for watercress.

BUTTERCRUNCH SALAD
1 head of buttercrunch lettuce
1 head of Boston lettuce
A few leaves of curly endive
½ cup grated raw beets

Tear the buttercrunch and Boston lettuces into bite-size pieces into the salad bowl. Cut the endive—it's harder to tear than the other lettuces. Toss together with basic dressing. Top with grated beets.

SUNBURST SALAD
small head of romaine
6 or 8 leaves of Boston lettuce
½ grated California carrot
½ grated raw beet
6 2-inch. slivers of raw yellow squash
½ ripe avocado
6 plum tomatoes

Break the lettuces into the salad bowl. Mound the grated carrot and beet in the center of the greens. Arrange the squash slivers star fashion from outside edge of grated vegetables to edge of bowl. Between the slivers place thin wedges of avocado. Tuck the tomatoes around the edge of the bowl at intervals. Drizzle basic dressing over all. Served with a side dish of fresh garden peas, this salad makes a meal and contains approximately the same number of calories as one serving of porterhouse steak.

Natural Dressings

The principles of making a natural dressing are simple. Use cold pressed oil (no other kind) and lemon juice instead of vinegar.

Skip salt and pepper. Vegetable powder (get it at your health store) may be used as a compromise.

BASIC DRESSING
2 tbsp. cold pressed oil
½ tsp. fresh lemon juice
1 tbsp. vegetable powder

This dressing is just about enough for one large salad and contains approximately 150 calories. The average mixed green salad will run about 100 calories, bringing your total average salad calorie count to 250. If you eat the salad without dressing you make a big saving. Just remember that these salads are designed as the main part of your meal—they can comprise the entire meal for either lunch or dinner.

AVOCADO DRESSING
¼ cup of cold pressed oil (I use safflower)
½ medium ripe avocado
1 stalk of celery
½ large green or red ripe pepper (or 1 small)
slice of Spanish onion

Blend together on high speed of blender. This is a natural that allows you to taste the subtle flavors of the salad greens without the stimulation of seasonings. If you're truly hungry it will taste delightful and will compliment your salad healthfully as well as tastefully. A half-cup of this dressing contains approximately 108 calories.

COTTAGE CHEESE DRESSING
2 tbsp. vegetable powder
¼ cup water
½ cup cottage cheese
1 stalk celery
¼ green pepper
1 medium ripe tomato

Blend ingredients together in blender. There are approximately 80 calories in ½ cup of this dressing.

TOMATO DRESSING
1 large ripe tomato
½ tbsp. safflower oil
½ green pepper

Blend together in blender. Contains approximately 100 calories.

You can use whichever dressing appeals to you on the various salads—make up your own combinations.

Finger salads are especially appetizing served with a few strips or chunks of unprocessed, low or unsalted cheese, like Jarlsberg Swiss, muenster, or farmer's. You can order unsalted, unpasteurized cheeses that are better for you and easier to digest, from the Kutter Cheese Co., Corfu, N.Y. (They'll send you a price list if you write to them.) If you don't have a weight problem, you can accompany finger salads with the fresh nuts of your choice.

Celery stalks are delicious stuffed with raw cashew butter from the health food store. Raw apple slices are delicious spread with it.

CHAPTER 13

Dynamic Natural Carbohydrate Recipes

Here are some of the Natural Carbohydrate recipes that have become favorites in our family over the years. Most are for our everyday meals, but some are designed for company dinners and special occasions.

Once you begin following these recipes you'll see how basically simple they are (less time for you in the kitchen!), and how easy it could be to create your own natural recipes.

As your body adapts itself to this simple, wonderfully satisfying way of eating, you'll learn instinctively how to maintain your correct weight and look your best. These recipes will help you get started.

Simple Soups to Make from Scratch

There are times, especially in cold weather, when nothing hits the spot like a hot bowl of soup. I'm including several surprisingly simple soup recipes for times like these. Notice that all the ingredients are fresh! Notice that you don't boil these soups! And notice that the first two take a mere ten minutes to make!

VEGETABLE SOUP

Wash and chop the entire leafy top from a bunch of fresh, hard celery. Dump into a stainless steel pot along with a pint of water and turn the heat on high. Add a cupful of chopped celery, a couple of cut up carrots (skin and all), and half a small onion, diced.

Whatever vegetables you have available can be diced and added to this mixture—green beans, broccoli, cauliflower, summer squash, green lima beans, or corn off the cob. Blend 4 or 5 fresh, ripe tomatoes at speed 2 or 3 for a minute. Dump this mixture into the pot. (If you can't get fresh, ripe tomatoes, use 2 cans stewed tomatoes.)

If the mixture seems too thick, add more water. When the soup comes to a boil, immediately turn the heat down and simmer with the lid on the pan for 10 minutes or so. Season to taste with Vegebase or other vegetable seasoning and a pinch of dill or tarragon. A pat of sweet butter or safflower margarine gives fuller flavor.

A bowl of this soup eaten before your big, green salad at night, and a helping of cottage cheese or 2 or 3 ounces of unprocessed cheese make a filling evening meal.

FRESH GREEN PEA SOUP
2 cups fresh green peas, or
   1 package frozen peas
½ cup half-and-half
¼ cup minced dried onions
1 tbsp. Vegebase

Steam peas until just tender, no more than 5 minutes. Put in blender with 2 cups boiling water. Add half-and-half, onion, and Vegebase or a pinch of Spike (another vegetable seasoning) to taste. Blend about a minute on high speed, then serve piping hot. You can garnish with a spoonful of grated cheese or ½ teaspoon of powdered raw nuts—walnuts or pecans.

With this recipe you can substitute fresh broccoli or celery for the green peas.

CREAMY CORN SOUP
3 ears of fresh corn, or
   ½ package frozen corn
1 small onion
¼ green pepper, minced
½ cup half-and-half
1 pint water
2 tbsp. Vegebase

If you're using fresh corn, scrape it off the cob with the dull edge of a knife to get the hearts of the kernels out of their pockets. Bring to a boil with the onion and pepper in a pint of pure water. Turn heat to low and simmer 5 minutes. Blend on high speed with the half-and-half until smooth. (The addition of a couple of tablespoons of natural cornmeal will make the soup even smoother.) Add Vegebase. Garnish with chopped parsley. Serves 2 to 3. If you're a weight-watcher, confine yourself to one small bowl of this soup. Have it for dinner with tossed green salad and steamed zucchini.

HEARTY BLACK BEAN SOUP
1 pound dried black beans
3 quarts water
¼ cup butter or peanut oil
3 tbsp. minced dried onion
Vegetable seasoning to taste
Chili powder (optional) to taste
¼ green pepper
¼ cup freshly grated parmesan
1 Spanish onion, sliced thin

Wash the beans and soak them in water overnight. Turn heat to high and when the beans begin to boil, turn the heat down to medium-low and simmer gently for 1½ to 2 hours, with lid ajar. (If the lid is tight, the liquid will bubble over.)

You may have to add water to the beans as they cook. When they're tender, ladle half of them, with some of the liquid and the dried minced onion, into the blender. Add the butter or oil and the seasoning and blend until smooth. Pour this back into the pan with the unblended beans. Add some water if necessary for proper consistency (the soup should be thick). Serve piping hot in pretty bowls, garnished with the minced green pepper, a tablespoon of freshly grated Parmesan cheese, and a thin slice of Spanish onion.

Vegetables and Casseroles

These dishes are a mainstay in your new way of eating. Cooked simply (if at all) but with a dash of imagination, dishes that feature vegetables can make eating a pleasure at the same time that they help you lose (or control) weight.

GREEN BEAN PATÉ
1 pound fresh green beans
6 ounces English walnuts
3 scallions
2 tbsp. cold pressed oil
1 tbsp. Vegebase
Pinch tarragon

Lightly steam the green beans. Place the walnuts in a wooden bowl and chop them coarsely with a double-bladed chopper. Add the beans and chop them in with the nuts. Add finely chopped scallions, green tops and all, to the walnut-bean mixture. Add the oil and Vegebase and mix everything together thoroughly. Add the tarragon. Serve in individual bowls; garnish with parsley and edge with diced ripe tomatoes. It could also be served on thick slices of ripe beefsteak tomatoes, garnished with thin rounds of red bell pepper and browned in a hot oven. This is a main dish to be eaten after the large salad. A good accompaniment is steamed cauliflower and asparagus spears.

BAKED STUFFED EGGPLANT
2 small eggplants
1 small Spanish onion
½ cup grated muenster cheese
2 tomatoes, chopped
1 tbsp. Vegebase and pinch of basil
2 tbsp. wheat germ

Place whole eggplants in steamer. Pour a cup of boiling water over them, place lid on pan and simmer about 15 minutes. Remove, allow to cool 5 minutes, and cut in half lengthwise. Scoop out and dice centers, saving the shells. Sauté onion with diced eggplant in a tablespoon of cold pressed oil. Add the tomatoes. Simmer for a minute, remove pan from heat and add the grated cheese, Vegebase, basil, and wheat germ. Spoon mixture back into shells, top with a square of muenster cheese and brown under the broiler until cheese begins to bubble. A good accompaniment to this dish would be steamed Brussels sprouts and yellow squash. Serves 2.

BROCCOLI CASSEROLE
1 large bunch fresh broccoli
1 small clove garlic, minced
¼ cup cold pressed oil
8 large mushrooms
8 ounces Finnish Swiss cheese
½ lemon

Lightly steam the broccoli until just tender and still bright green. In separate small pan cook the garlic in the oil until yellow but not brown. Remove from heat and add the juice of the half lemon and a small amount of vegetable seasoning. Arrange broccoli spears in a baking dish. Arrange mushroom slices attractively around sides of dish. Drizzle the garlic and lemon mixture evenly over the broccoli and top with grated Swiss cheese. Sprinkle with paprika and some dried vegetables. Heat in the oven until the cheese begins to bubble. Serve immediately. This casserole, which serves 2 generously, makes a good evening meal with steamed green beans or zucchini and, as always, a large salad.

SQUASH À LA JOY
4 small, tender yellow squash or young zucchini
1 small Spanish onion, peeled and quartered
2 tbsp. Vegebase
2 tbsp. sweet butter or safflower margarine

Steam the squash and onion until barely tender—about 5 to 7 minutes. Put half the squash, along with its juices, into the blender. Add other ingredients. Blend on high speed for just a minute. Mash the remaining squash with a potato masher or fork. Pour blended squash over the mashed squash. Sprinkle with a pinch of tarragon and serve at once. Serves 2 generously.

EGGPLANT STEAK
1 medium eggplant
Cold pressed oil
2 large ripe tomatoes
8 ounces mozzarella or muenster cheese
Vegebase and oregano to taste

Cut eggplant into thick slices. Brush each side generously with oil, lay slices close together on a baking sheet, and brown on each side under the broiler.

Arrange eggplant slices in the bottom of a shallow baking dish. Top each slice with a thick slice of tomato, a thick slice of cheese, and a sprinkling of Vegebase and oregano. Pop into a 450° oven for 10 minutes, or until the cheese begins to bubble and brown.

STUFFED ZUCCHINI (OR EGGPLANT)
1 large zucchini squash or eggplant
2 tbsp. safflower oil
2 medium-sized tomatoes, ripe and red
2 cups Polly-O ricotta cheese
4 ounces grated mozzarella

Slice the zucchini or eggplant on the round. Lightly brush each slice, front and back, with safflower oil. Place on a baking sheet and put under the broiler until lightly browned on each side. (Total browning time about 5 minutes.) In a safflower-oiled baking dish, place a layer of sliced tomatoes, a layer of the zucchini or eggplant slices, and a layer of ricotta cheese, sprinkled with mozzarella. Repeat. On top of the final layer sprinkle a couple of pinches of fresh or dried basil, and, if you wish, a teaspoon of Vegebase. Put in the oven and bake at 400 degrees until it begins to bubble around the edges—usually, 10 or 15 minutes. Serve hot. This recipe serves 4. It's easy to make two small casseroles and freeze the extra one, well-covered, for future use.

CHEESE-TOPPED CAULIFLOWER
1 small head cauliflower
6 oz. unprocessed cheese (Kutter, muenster, mozzarella, or Swiss)
Watercress for garnishing

Steam the cauliflower whole, until just tender, in a pan it just fits in. (About 15 minutes. Takes longer because it's whole.) Quickly lift the lid and put the two slices of cheese crisscross over the top of the cauliflower. Put the lid back on. Take off the heating unit; let stand for 5 minutes. Transfer whole cauliflower to serving dish. Sprinkle lightly with paprika and encircle with fresh watercress. Serve at once.

LENTIL STEW
1 cup dried lentils
1 small sweet onion, chopped
½ green bell pepper, diced
1 quart water
2 or 3 ripe tomatoes, blended
Vegetable seasoning to taste
Pinch of dried dill weed
1 tsp. safflower margarine, or
    sweet butter

Put lentils, onion, and pepper into pot of rapidly boiling water. Immediately turn heat to simmer, place lid on pan, and steam until lentils are tender—about 30 minutes. They're done when they mash easily with a fork. Test during steaming. If lentils get dry, add another cup or two of water. When done, add the blended tomatoes (use stewed tomatoes if you can't get good fresh ones), dill weed, and margarine or butter. Add Vegebase or other vegetable seasoning sparingly. Since this recipe serves 4 generously, you can freeze what's left.

DEBBIE'S VEGETABLE MEDLEY

½ stalk of green celery
½ fresh carrot
¼ Spanish onion
6 oz. frozen Chinese pea pods
6 large dried black mushrooms
1 cup sprouts, either mung or alfalfa
1 tbsp. safflower oil

Put oil into heavy stainless steel skillet or pan, on high heat unit. As it heats up, add celery, which you've cut into one-inch slivers, and the carrot, onion, and the pea pods and black mushrooms, which you've broken into pieces. When the vegetables are sizzling nicely, put the lid on and turn the heat off. Shake the pan a couple of times during the 5 minutes you allow the steam to tenderize the vegetables. Remove the lid, add mung beans, and replace lid, letting the warmth from the pan heat up the sprouts. Sprinkle lightly with a whisper of vegetable seasoning—Vegebase or Spike—and serve immediately with Fluffy Brown Rice (see below).

Grains

Some people (I'm one of them) find it easy to overdo—and gain weight—on grain foods. If you are a weight watcher, then watch your grains! (You'll see that I've included only moderate amounts of grain foods in my Month of Menus.)

FLUFFY BROWN RICE

3 cups water
1 cup brown rice
1 tbsp. vegetable seasoning

Bring water to a boil and add rice. Cover and reduce heat to a simmer for 15 or 20 minutes, until tender.

WILD AND WONDERFUL RICE

4 cups cold water
1 cup long grain brown rice
¼ cup wild rice
1 tbsp. oil
1 small Spanish onion
12 large mushrooms
1 tsp. vegetable seasoning

Put water in a two-quart saucepan and bring to a boil over high heat. Add both kinds of rice. Turn heat down to simmer, place lid on pan, and allow to simmer for 30 minutes or until tender.

While rice is steaming, sauté one small Spanish onion and a dozen large, chopped mushrooms in a skillet. Season with Vegebase. Serve the rice topped with the onions and mushrooms. Makes a filling company dish or simply a main dish to be eaten after the evening salad and accompanied by another steamed vegetable such as summer squash or steamed broccoli.

SPANISH CASSEROLE
1 cup mixed brown and wild rice
1 cup light cream mixed with ½ cup water
1 medium zucchini squash, sliced (yellow crookneck squash or eggplant may be substituted)
1 large potato, well-scrubbed and sliced
1 Spanish onion, thinly sliced
1 green pepper, cut in strips
Vegebase
¼ tsp. dried tarragon
¼ tsp. dried basil
Butter or soy margarine

Spread the rice in the bottom of a three-quart baking dish. Pour half the cream-water mixture over it. Alternate layers of zucchini, potato, onion, and pepper, sprinkling each layer with vegetable seasoning, tarragon, and basil. End with a layer of squash, sprinkled with Vegebase. Pour remaining liquid mixture over all, dot with butter or soy margarine, and bake uncovered in a 425° oven for an hour, or until tender when tested with a fork.

ZESTY KASHA CASSEROLE
1 tbsp. Herbemare
2 cups water
1 cup medium or coarse kasha (buckwheat groats)
½ cup light cream

Topping:
½ Spanish onion, diced
1 cup diced celery
¼ cup green pepper, diced
1 small carrot, grated
1 cup raw green beans, cut
2 tbsp. cold pressed oil
2 tbsp. Vegebase

Add Herbemare to water and bring to boil. Add kasha, turn heat off completely, replace lid and allow to sit, covered, for 25 to 30 minutes.

While you're waiting, sauté the vegetables in oil and add a dash of vegetable seasoning. Uncover the kasha, add cream, and mix lightly with a fork. The idea is to keep the kasha light and fluffy, each grain separate.

Spread the kasha in an oiled baking dish, spread vegetable mixture on top, sprinkle lightly with Vegebase and dot with butter. Place in a hot oven (425°) until top begins to brown. Serve at once.

(*Note:* Millet, a light, delicious, and under-appreciated grain, can be substituted for kasha in this recipe.)

FRESH SWEET CORN, KENTUCKY STYLE

2 ears fresh sweet corn
¼ large Spanish onion
¼ fresh green pepper, diced
1 tbsp. sweet butter, safflower margarine or oil

Husk the corn. Place a large bowl in the sink and holding the corn over the bowl, cut the kernels off the cob with a sharp knife, cutting in an upward motion. Cut just the tips off the kernels; then swing the back, or dull edge of the knife in a downward motion, removing the hearts and juice of the remainder of the cut kernels. (Go over the cob twice to be sure to remove all the hearts.)

Place a one-quart skillet over high heat and brown the onion and pepper in the oil or margarine. Add the corn, stir, then put lid on and turn heat off. Let sit for 5 minutes and serve.

DELICIOUS WHOLE-WHEAT LINGUINE

3 quarts water
1 8-ounce pkg. whole-wheat linguine (from your health food store)
4 tbsp. cold pressed oil, or butter
1 clove fresh garlic, finely minced
Vegetable seasoning to taste

Bring water to a rapid boil, add linguine, and boil until strands are barely soft (*al dente*). Meanwhile, in butter or oil, lightly brown garlic. Drain the linguine and toss with the oil- or butter-and-garlic mixture; add vegetable seasoning. Serve as the main dish with a large green salad and a succulent vegetable, such as summer squash.

Fresh Fruits

Fresh, ripe fruit is best when eaten whole. If sliced, it should be cut into large slices immediately before serving and sliced further as you eat it, when feasible, since vitamins are lost through oxidation when cut fruits are exposed to the air.

FRESH FRUIT SPECIAL
2 or 3 leaves Boston *or* buttercrunch lettuce
2 cups fresh, cubed pineapple
½ cup fresh blueberries
1 small ripe papaya, sliced
4 large fresh strawberries
½ cup cottage cheese
2 shelled walnut halves

Arrange lettuce leaves on luncheon plate. In the center of the plate make a mound of the pineapple chunks. Arrange blueberries, papaya slices, and strawberries around the edge. Spoon the dry cottage cheese right in the center of the pineapple. Garnish with the walnut halves.

This makes a deliciously satisfying lunch. In case you're wondering about the calorie count, it adds up to 528—less than what you'd get in a peanut-butter-and-jelly sandwich.

PINEAPPLE DELIGHT
½ fresh Hawaiian pineapple
1 medium-sized navel orange
5 or 6 crisp, dark green romaine lettuce leaves
1 generous scoop *uncreamed* cottage cheese, or
    farmer's cheese
2 shelled pecan halves
Small sprig fresh green parsley

Peel and core pineapple and slice lengthwise into strips. Peel and section orange. Arrange lettuce leaves on one of your prettiest luncheon plates. Arrange slices of pineapple and orange sections on the lettuce leaves. Top with cottage cheese and garnish with parsley and sliced pecan halves. (Garnishes are to be eaten!)

MANGO DIVINE
Cut a medium-sized mango in half, slicing over the large, flat seed on both sides. With a sharp paring knife score the meat of the mango in cubes without cutting through the skin. Invert the two halves and arrange on an oval plate, along with some bing cherries

and small bunches of white seedless grapes. Mango Divine is a meal in itself. It's not only tempting to look at but delicious and nutritious.

APRICOT FLUFF
4 ounces unsulphured, dried apricots
4 ounces pitted Khadrawi dates
4 ounces plain *or* vanilla yogurt
2 ounces date sugar
Sprig mint

Soak apricots in water to cover overnight. Add dates to this mixture and blend at high speed (you may have to add a little more water to avoid straining the motor). Pour the fluff into individual stemmed dessert glasses. Spoon yogurt over the top, sprinkle with date sugar (from the health food store) and garnish with a sprig of mint.

This makes an elegant breakfast. You could also have it for lunch, along with a ripe banana, or half a mango, or a large, juicy ripe peach or pear. One serving of Apricot Fluff and a banana contains fewer calories than a slice of pound cake.

Nut Butters

As a part of your protein for either breakfast, lunch, or dinner, fresh, raw nut butters are delicious. Don't think of them as an accompaniment to bread or crackers; spread them on sliced apples, or celery, or even strawberries.

BASIC NUT BUTTER RECIPE
2 cups raw nuts (either cashews, walnuts, almonds, *or*
    sunflower or pumpkin seeds)
2 or 3 tbsp. cold pressed safflower *or* peanut oil

Blend nuts to a powder in your blender. Add oil through the top of the blender, stopping the motor once or twice to push the mixture off the sides.

This recipe makes about a cup of nut butter. Store it covered in a glass or clear plastic container.

Drinks

Healthful fruit or vegetable drinks make refreshing treats, midmorning or midafternoon. The Green Goddess (below) is special, however, in that it's super-energizing and high in amino acid content. You can make it for yourself several times a week.

GREEN GODDESS
Small bunch fresh parsley
4 or 5 stalks celery
15 or 20 crisp spinach leaves (optional)

Separate parsley into 4 or 5 small bunches and push each bunch through a juice extractor with a piece of the celery. Drink this jade-colored energizer immediately, as it will oxidize and begin losing its precious vitamins if you let it sit around.

TROPICAL TREAT
1 fresh Hawaiian pineapple

Halve, peel, and slice the pineapple lengthwise; then push it through a juice extractor. (I use an Acme, which I bought in a health food store.)

For me this heavenly drink plus a few seeds or nuts or a scoop of cottage cheese make a delightful lunch. It's also a good way to start the day if you're a person who does better having breakfast.

CARROT JUICE
2 large or 3 or 4 small carrots

Thinly peel carrots and feed them into the juicer. (If you're using large carrots, slice them in half.) For a less sweet drink, feed 2 or 3 celery stalks into the juicer as well.

Drink 15 or 30 minutes before the noon or evening meal; this drink will take the edge off your appetite.

BANANA MILK SHAKE
2 frozen very ripe bananas
8 ounces milk (certified raw, if available)

Blend ingredients together until frothy. Pour into tall, slim glasses, sprinkle with a dash of nutmeg, and enjoy.

(*Note:* You may use unfrozen bananas if you toss two or three ice cubes into the blender with them.)

This drink, with a piece of fresh fruit, makes a healthy meal-in-a-glass for the children.

PINEAPPLE COOLER
8 oz. unsweetened pineapple juice
A thin shaving of lemon rind
2 or 3 ice cubes

Blend ingredients together on high speed in the blender and pour into tall glasses. Makes a refreshing drink to serve guests or family on a warm summer afternoon.

Special Recipes and Suggestions for Entertaining

Following are some delightful dishes to serve guests or even, on special occasions, the family. They will not help you lose (or control) weight but these recipes are all based on good, natural foods. You can feel secure, as you entertain, that what you're serving is both healthful and delicious. Friends have said they feel special and well taken care of when they come to our house!

HORS D'OEUVRES

"Having drinks" is a well-ensconced American social custom. When you invite friends for dinner they will expect to spend some time relaxing with a drink and some appetizers before the meal. Here's what you can serve them.

SOUR CREAM AND COTTAGE CHEESE DIP

8 oz. sour cream
1 cup uncreamed cottage cheese (small curd)
2 tbsp. Vegebase
2 tbsp. minced dried onion
½ green pepper, grated
1 tsp. dried dill

Mix these ingredients together and put in a pretty bowl, garnished with crisp leaves of watercress. Sprinkle a dash of paprika in the center. Place the bowl in the center of a large round tray or platter. Around the bowl arrange, in neat sections, whole small tomatoes, crisp green celery sticks, carrot sticks, cauliflower florets, and strips of raw green pepper.

STUFFED MUSHROOMS

12 large white fresh mushrooms
¼ Spanish onion
¼ cup butter
¾ cup whole-wheat breadcrumbs
¼ cup cream
1 tsp. Herbemare
Oregano to taste

Wash mushrooms; pat dry and remove stems. Chop the stems and onion and sauté in the butter until the onions are translucent. Add breadcrumbs, cream, and Herbemare. Spoon the mixture into the mushroom caps, arrange in a baking dish, sprinkle lightly with oregano. Pop into a 450° oven for 10 minutes, or until tops begin to brown nicely. Serve immediately.

CHEESE TRAY WITH CRACKERS

Trim the rind from a large wedge of Jarlsberg cheese and set on a decorative ceramic or wooden cheese board with a cheese knife. Accompany with a bowl of well-drained, jumbo black olives and a basket filled with whole-wheat Venus wafers, swedish rye thins, or rice wafers.

APPLES AND MOZZARELLA CHEESE

Peel and thickly slice 2 apples. In the center of a small platter arrange quarter-inch slices of fresh mozzarella (try an Italian cheese store for this). Arrange the apple slices in a circle at the outside of the platter. Garnish with sprigs of parsley.

DRINKS

I keep bottled tomato juice, unsweetened pineapple juice, and apple juice on hand, as well as chilled Perrier and a bottle or two of white wine, for guests.

CHEESE CASSEROLE

(*This dish must be prepared the night before you serve it.*)
¼ cup safflower margarine or sweet butter, melted
½ loaf sliced whole-wheat bread, cubed
4 ounces natural Cheddar cheese, cubed
½ Spanish onion, diced
½ green pepper, grated
1 tbsp. Spike
1 tbsp. Vegebase
1 pint milk (raw if you can get it)
3 fertile eggs, country grown (if you can get them)

Oil a two-quart casserole dish with safflower oil. Mix the bread cubes, cheese, onion, pepper, and seasonings in a large bowl. Put the milk in the blender with the eggs and run on high speed for about a minute, or until frothy. Pour the milk and eggs over the above mixture and place in prepared casserole dish. Drizzle with melted butter, cover tightly, and let sit overnight in the refrigerator. Before serving, take the casserole out of the fridge. Pop it into the oven, uncovered, and bake for approximately 35 to 40 minutes, or until it is lightly browned and puffy looking on top. Serve immediately, as the main course, in lieu of roast beef!

WHOLE-WHEAT LASAGNA
8 ounces of whole-wheat lasagna noodles
1 farm-grown fertile egg
2 or 3 tbsp. half-and-half
16 ounces of Polly-O ricotta cheese
Pinch Vegebase
Special tomato sauce (recipe follows)
8 large slices mozzarella cheese
8 ounces freshly grated Parmesan cheese

Boil the noodles in a large stainless steel pot in 4 quarts of water. Add a tablespoon of safflower oil to the boiling water. Boil for 10 minutes, or until noodles are tender. (Whole-wheat noodles will be firmer than regular ones so don't overcook.) Drain the noodles in a colander, separate them, and lay them out on a dry terry towel. Beat the egg and half-and-half into the ricotta with an electric mixer until it's light and fluffy. Season with a pinch or two of Vegebase. In a two-quart casserole, spoon a layer of sauce, a layer of slightly overlapping noodles, a layer of ricotta cheese, mozzarella cheese, and Parmesan. Repeat the layering, ending up with a top layer of sauce. Bake in a preheated 425° oven for approximately half an hour, or until it's bubbling nicely and filling the house with delectable smells. This dish should be taken out and allowed to cool and set for at least half an hour before serving, so it won't be too gooey when you serve it. (Recipe serves 6 generously.)

SPECIAL SAUCE
12 large, juicy, vine-ripened tomatoes
¼ cup imported olive oil
2 large cloves of fresh garlic
1 tbsp. Herbemare
1 tbsp. Vegebase
1 tsp. dried basil (I grow my own and freeze it for winter use.)

Core and quarter tomatoes and put them in the blender in batches, using a low speed, to barely macerate them. Yellow the minced garlic in the oil in a two-quart stainless steel pan. Add tomatoes and heat until bubbling. Add the seasonings, then turn heat to low and allow to simmer gently, uncovered, for 15 or 20 minutes.

Desserts

As you will see when you switch over to them, natural desserts are the most luscious there are. They *can* be high in calories, however. A word to the wise!

TROPICAL SURPRISE ICE CREAM
1 large ripe mango
12 pitted soft dates
1 cup chilled heavy cream
½ tsp. lemon juice

Peel mango and cut the meat from the seed. Blend, with dates, on medium speed, until fruit is mushy. Pour cream into a chilled mixing bowl, add lemon juice, and whip until it forms soft peaks. Fold cream into the date-mango mixture and turn into ice cube tray. Freeze, stirring twice with a fork during the freezing process. (Bananas or ripe peaches may be substituted for the mangoes.)

FIVE-FRUIT SUNDAE
2 cups seedless white grapes
2 cups fresh ripe strawberries
1 cup ripe blueberries
1 can drained, unsweetened pineapple chunks
½ pound fresh, soft ricotta cheese
Date sugar
4 fresh red cherries, pitted

Gently mix the fruit together in a large bowl (except the cherries). Spoon into sundae glasses, filling them ⅔ full. Top each with a scoop of ricotta cheese, sprinkle with a teaspoon of date sugar, and garnish with a cherry.

This makes a good company or bridge dessert. It's also a nice lunch. What an alternative to the hot fudge sundae!

NATURALLY SWEET DREAM DESSERT
1 cup heavy cream
20 soft dates
2 very ripe bananas

Quickly blend together in blender the cream and 16 of the dates. Set out 4 stemmed compote glasses. Slice half a banana into each; top with date mixture and decorate with date pieces from the remaining four dates. Can be made ahead and stored, covered, in the refrigerator.

BANANA-COCONUT CREAM PIE

1 16-oz. package soft pitted dates
4 very ripe bananas
1 cup cream
1 20-oz. can unsweetened pineapple, drained
½ cup unsweetened shredded coconut

Press dates down flat in the bottom of a glass pie pan. Slice the bananas on in an even layer. Pour on top of that the cream and pineapple that have been blended together in the blender. Sprinkle generously with the shredded coconut. Cover the top with plastic wrap and chill for 2 or 3 hours before serving.

FRESH FRUIT AMBROSIA

2 cups ripe Hawaiian or canned unsweetened pineapple chunks
1 cup fresh blueberries
½ cup fresh strawberries, halved
1 cup plain or vanilla yogurt
1 tbsp. slivered almonds.

Combine fruits in a bowl. Top with yogurt and sprinkle with slivered almonds.

Lunch Suggestions for the Family

PITACADO

¼ ripe avocado
1 whole-wheat pita (round Syrian bread)
1 tsp. minced sweet onion
½ cup fresh alfalfa sprouts
¼ cup grated bell pepper
½ cup finely slivered green lettuce

Mash the avocado. Fill the inside of the pita with the layered up vegetables. Eat slowly and relish. This is good eaten with a large stalk of crisp green celery.

RICA-DOG

This is my answer to the hot dog. Try it. Maybe you'll start a new trend among the young set around your house!

2 large dark green leaves romaine
½ cup Polly-O ricotta cheese
½ ripe tomato
¼ cup alfalfa sprouts
1 tsp. finely minced sweet onion or chives
A light sprinkling of Vegebase

Set the two romaine leaves on top of each other, end to top, so that there's nice fullness at both ends. Spread the ricotta evenly along the rib of the lettuce. Slice tomato into five flat slices and stagger them along the length of the leaf, on top of the ricotta. Spread the onion on top of the tomato slices, and the sprouts on top of that. Sprinkle lightly with Vegebase. Roll the lettuce over all, sort of wrapping it all up. Serve on a sturdy paper napkin or paper towel, with an extra napkin or towel for sanitary reasons. I think nothing of eating two of these and calling it lunch!

By the way, you can get a Vege-shaker (similar to a sugar-shaker but with the right-size slits to allow a free dispensation of Vegebase) by ordering from the *Shangri-La Natural Hygiene Institute, Bonita Springs, Florida, 33923*. They'll send you a price list upon request.

CHAPTER 14

A Month of Born-Again Menus with Calorie and Protein Count

You'll notice that the menus I have included tally up at slightly under 1200 calories a day. If you follow the plan faithfully you should be able to lose weight. If you follow the 30-Day Born-Again Body Program (Chapter 18), which refers you back to these menus and which also includes plenty of exercise and two short fasts, you can lose anywhere from five to twenty pounds in a month, depending upon your metabolism.

If you have a weight problem you'll get those unwanted pounds off more easily if you forget about eating breakfast—providing, of course, that you don't make up for it by overeating at lunch and dinner.

If you don't have a weight problem you may add nuts or seeds to those breakfasts that don't already include them. You may also have larger portions of starch and concentrated protein and fat foods if you feel hungry for them.

If you are accustomed to having a hot drink such as coffee and need help getting away from it, get a container of Pero, a coffee substitute, and have that instead. You'll find it at your favorite special food or health food shop. Have it before your breakfast (if you like) and after your evening meal. You may also substitute cynopep, an herb tea combination of mint and rose hips.

If you find complete abstinence from meat too difficult to manage initially, substitute fresh fish twice a week for the main course at dinner instead of the baked potato, rice, or casserole dish.

You may also substitute poached or soft-boiled egg for nuts or seeds once a week at breakfast.

In adapting these menus to your own metabolism it's important to remember that no two persons' bodies function in quite the same way. Your needs are different from mine. Your metabolism may be set at a higher speed, or a lower one. You need to adjust these menus to fit your particular body. Try them, carefully observe the results, and then decide for yourself whether you need larger portions of some foods and smaller portions of others, or whether you do best having your large meal at noon or at night.

(*Note:* For those of you who feel you cannot make the switch to total vegetarianism all at once, the following fish and/or egg substitutions may be made in your "Month of Menus.")

Week One

TUESDAY:

At breakfast, skip the Brazil nuts, which are high in protein, and have an extra orange or grapefruit. Then, for dinner, you may substitute five ounces of broiled swordfish for the Broccoli Casserole.

THURSDAY:

At lunch, instead of the cottage cheese, you may have a two-egg omelet seasoned with herbs.

SATURDAY:

At lunch you may have four ounces of broiled shrimp seasoned with some lemon juice or vegetable seasoning instead of the ricotta cheese.

Week Two

SUNDAY:

At dinner you may substitute three ounces of baked shad for the potato.

WEDNESDAY:

At dinner you may substitute three ounces of broiled bluefish for the potato.

SATURDAY:

For lunch you may substitute two eggs scrambled in a teaspoon of butter for the baked apple and cottage cheese.

Week Three

TUESDAY:

At dinner you may have ¼ pound filet of flounder, either poached or broiled, instead of the baked potato.

THURSDAY:

At breakfast you may substitute one poached, boiled, or scrambled egg for the pecans.

SATURDAY:

At dinner you may have three ounces of broiled fish of your choice instead of stuffed eggplant.

Week Four

TUESDAY:

At lunch you may substitute two scrambled eggs and a small green salad for the Fresh Fruit Special.

THURSDAY:

At lunch you may have one scoop of tuna salad on lettuce, garnished with fresh tomato wedges, and 8 stalks of steamed asparagus instead of the Fresh Fruit Special.

SUNDAY:

At dinner you may substitute three ounces of broiled or poached red snapper for the Lentil Stew.

Menus to Help You Get Started

FIRST WEEK

MONDAY

Breakfast:		Calories	Protein Grams
1 whole ripe cantaloupe		160	4.0
Lunch:			
Fruit Plate:			
1 bunch of white grapes		100	1.0
10 cherries		45	1.0
3 nectarines		150	3.0
½ cup cottage cheese		117	14.0
	Total	**412**	**19.0**
Dinner:			
Super-sized Mixed Green Salad* with			
zesty Basic Dressing		305	13.5
1 baked potato, 1 pat butter**		180	4.0
½ cup green beans		15	1.0
½ cup lima beans		85	5.0
	Total	**585**	**23.5**
Snack:			
1 large apple		80	trace
3 dried figs		168	2.7
	Total	**248**	**2.7**
	Daily Total	**1405**	**49.2**

TUESDAY

Breakfast:		Calories	Protein Grams
Large grapefruit		100	2.0
8 Brazil nuts·		185	4.0
	Total	**285**	**6.0**
Lunch:			
3 juicy ripe peaches		120	3.0
1 sugary ripe papaya		156	2.4
1 large ripe banana		100	1.0
	Total	**376**	**6.4**

* All salads are meant to be super-sized, almost a meal-in-a-bowl.
** Sweet butter is recommended.

Dinner:

Huge Rainbow Salad	218	17.2
Large portion cheese-topped Broccoli Casserole	274	12.4
1 cup steamed green peas	110	8.0
Total	**602**	**37.6**

Snack:

1 pear	100	1.0
Daily Total	**1363**	**51.0**

WEDNESDAY

Breakfast:	*Calories*	*Protein Grams*
2 oranges	130	2.0
1 ounce sunflower seeds	160	4.0
Total	**290**	**6.0**

Lunch:

Fresh Fruit Ambrosia with yogurt and almonds	460	15.0

Dinner:

Crunchy Finger Salad with ½ cup rich Avocado Dressing	236	8.6
1 golden baked acorn squash, 1 pat butter	165	4.0
1 cup succulent steamed zucchini	30	2.0
Total	**431**	**14.6**

Snack:

1 sugar-ripe peach	40	1.0
Daily Total	**1221**	**36.6**

THURSDAY

Breakfast:	*Calories*	*Protein Grams*
½ fresh pineapple	140	0.5

Lunch:

Watercress Special	170	5.7
½ cup cottage cheese	117	14.0
2 beefsteak tomatoes	66	3.2
Total	**353**	**22.9**

Dinner:

		Calories	Protein Grams
Giant Mixed Green Salad		155	13.5
1 ripe avocado		370	5.0
1 cup summer squash		30	2.0
6 large asparagus spears		15	1.5
with 1 tsp. melted butter		35	trace
	Total	**605**	**22.0**

Snack:

1 average-sized apple		70	trace
	Daily Total	**1168**	**45.4**

FRIDAY

Breakfast:		*Calories*	*Protein Grams*
1 large watermelon wedge		110	2.0

Lunch:

1½ cups Vegetable Soup		180	4.0
2 crunchy celery stalks stuffed with 2 tbsp. natural peanut butter		200	8.0
	Total	**380**	**12.0**

Dinner:

Super-sized Mixed Vegetable Salad		269	21.0
1 ear hot corn on the cob with 1 pat butter		105	2.0
1 cup sliced steamed beets		55	2.0
	Total	**429**	**25.0**

Snack:

6 natural dates		132	1.2
	Daily Total	**1051**	**40.2**

SATURDAY

Breakfast:		*Calories*	*Protein Grams*
1 sugar-sweet papaya		156	2.4
1 ounce sunflower seeds		160	4.0
	Total	**316**	**6.4**

Lunch:

2 beefsteak tomatoes		66	3.2
2 stalks green celery		10	trace
½ green pepper, cut in strips		11	0.6
⅔ cup ricotta cheese		219	19.0
	Total	**306**	**22.8**

Dinner:

Large Super Sprout salad with Basic Dressing		305	12.0
1 baked yam with 1 pat butter		176	2.0
12 whole steamed green beans		15	1.0
1 cup buttered Brussels sprouts		90	7.0
	Total	**586**	**22.0**

Snack:

1 soft ripe persimmon		96	0.9
	Daily Total	**1304**	**52.1**

SUNDAY

Breakfast:	*Calories*	*Protein Grams*
½ large ripe Spanish melon	120	1.4

Lunch:

Fruit basket:			
2 ripe pears		200	2.0
1 cup red-ripe bing cherries		105	2.0
6 dates		132	1.2
2 ripe fresh figs		60	0.9
	Total	**497**	**6.1**

Dinner:

Giant-sized Spinach Salad with Basic Dressing		262	18.5
Small portion Zesty Kasha Casserole		135	2.6
1 cup steamed kale		45	5.0
1 cup steamed carrots		50	1.0
	Total	**492**	**27.1**

Snack:

1 large bunch of grapes		100	1.0
	Daily Total	**1209**	**35.6**

SECOND WEEK

MONDAY

Breakfast:	*Calories*	*Protein Grams*
3 sugar-ripe peaches	120	3.0
1 cup fresh blueberries	90	1.0

	Total	**210**	**4.0**

Lunch:

1 cup steaming Celery Soup		130	0.8
Large Watercress Special		170	5.7
10 almonds		60	6.0
	Total	**360**	**12.5**

Dinner:

Huge Rainbow Salad with Basic Dressing	368	17.2
Medium serving Spanish Casserole	213	3.8
1 cup steamed green peas	110	8.0
Total	**691**	**29.0**
Daily Total	**1261**	**45.5**

TUESDAY

Breakfast:	*Calories*	*Protein Grams*
1 pint fresh ripe strawberries	110	2.0
8 raw cashews	88	5.0
Total	**198**	**7.0**

Lunch:

3 beefsteak tomatoes	99	4.8
½ cup cottage cheese	117	14.0
1 cup steamed whole green beans	30	2.0
Total	**246**	**20.8**

Dinner:

½ recipe Debbie's Vegetable Medley	107	4.2
1 cup Wild and Wonderful Rice, 1 pat butter	213	3.8
Very large Mixed Green Salad, Basic Dressing included	305	13.5
Total	**625**	**21.5**

Snack:

1 large ripe banana	100	1.0
Daily Total	**1169**	**50.3**

WEDNESDAY

Breakfast:	*Calories*	*Protein Grams*
1 whole ripe cantaloupe	160	4.0

Lunch:

½ recipe Fresh Fruit Special	264	10.2
1 bunch of white grapes	100	1.0
10 fresh cherries	45	1.0
Total	**409**	**12.2**

Dinner:

1 large bowl Vegetable Soup	240	4.0
Huge Rainbow Salad, Basic Dressing included	368	17.2
1 baked potato, 1 pat butter	180	4.0
Total	**788**	**25.2**

Snack:

1 orange	65	1.0
Daily Total	**1422**	**42.4**

THURSDAY

Breakfast:		*Calories*	*Protein Grams*
2 oranges		130	2.0
2 tbsp. pignolias		84	2.0
	Total	**214**	**4.0**
Lunch:			
Mixed Green Salad		155	13.5
2 slices whole-wheat bread, ½ pat butter each slice		155	6.0
	Total	**310**	**19.5**
Dinner:			
2 cups Creamy Corn Soup		230	5.0
Giant-sized Super Sprouts salad		155	12.0
1 cup steamed kale		45	5.0
½ cup steamed fresh carrots		25	.5
	Total	**455**	**24.0**
Snack:			
1 cup blueberries		90	1.0
	Daily Total	**1069**	**48.5**

FRIDAY

Breakfast:		*Calories*	*Protein Grams*
Frothy Pineapple Perfection		140	1.0
1 cup blueberries		90	1.0
	Total	**230**	**2.0**
Lunch:			
1 bowl Fresh Green Pea Soup		200	8.7
2 celery stalks		10	trace
½ green pepper, cut in strips		11	0.6
2 rye thins		45	2.0
	Total	**266**	**11.3**
Dinner:			
Large crisp Spinach and Mushroom Salad with Basic Dressing		262	18.5
Large portion Baked Stuffed Eggplant		375	11.8
1 steamed artichoke with butter and lemon		64	2.8
	Total	**701**	**33.1**
	Daily Total	**1197**	**46.4**

SATURDAY

Breakfast:		Calories	Protein Grams
1 whole honeydew melon		500	10.0
Lunch:			
2 baked apples		140	0.6
½ cup cottage cheese		117	14.0
	Total	**257**	**14.6**
Dinner:			
Gigantic Buttercrunch Salad with Basic Dressing		260	9.0
1 large baked potato, 2 pats butter		215	4.0
6 large spears steamed broccoli		60	6.0
	Total	**535**	**19.0**
Snack:			
1 orange		65	1.0
15 English walnut halves		98	6.0
	Total	**163**	**7.0**
	Daily Total	**1455**	**50.6**

SUNDAY

Breakfast:		Calories	Protein Grams
1 grapefruit		100	2.0
12 pecan halves		81	1.1
	Total	**181**	**3.1**
Lunch:			
Fruit basket:			
4 ripe nectarines		200	4.0
½ fresh pineapple		140	0.5
1 bunch of grapes		100	1.0
6 leaves romaine lettuce		10	1.0
	Total	**450**	**6.5**
Dinner:			
Large Mixed Green Salad, Basic Dressing included		305	13.5
¼ recipe Cheese-Topped Cauliflower		76	7.8
1 cup steamed green lima beans		170	10.0
	Total	**551**	**31.3**
Snack:			
2 stalks green celery		10	trace
	Daily Total	**1192**	**40.9**

THIRD WEEK

MONDAY

Breakfast:		Calories	Protein Grams
2 oranges		130	2.0
15 almonds		90	9.0
	Total	220	11.0

Lunch:	Calories	Protein Grams
Mango Divine—meal on a plate!	245	4.4

Dinner:		Calories	Protein Grams
Huge Rainbow Salad, Basic Dressing included		368	17.2
2 slices whole rye bread, buttered		190	4.0
1 cup steamed escarole		46	3.9
½ recipe Squash à la Joy		148	2.4
	Total	752	27.5
	Daily Total	1217	42.9

TUESDAY

Breakfast:	Calories	Protein Grams
1 large wedge watermelon	110	2.0

Lunch:		Calories	Protein Grams
Apricot Yogurt Fluff spooned over a large ripe peach		226	4.6
1 cup fresh blueberries		90	1.0
	Total	316	5.6

Dinner:		Calories	Protein Grams
Large Finger Salad without the tomato, ½ cup Avocado Dressing		205	7.6
Medium portion Zesty Kasha Casserole		190	3.0
1 cup sliced steamed beets		55	2.0
1 cup green peas		110	8.0
	Total	560	20.6

Snack:		Calories	Protein Grams
2 stalks celery stuffed with 1 ounce muenster cheese		103	6.2
	Daily Total	1089	34.4

WEDNESDAY

Breakfast:		Calories	Protein Grams
Green Goddess drink		36	3.0
15 filberts		98	3.2
	Total	134	6.2

Lunch:			
1 whole papaya		156	2.4
1 cup raspberries		70	1.0
8 fresh figs		240	3.6
	Total	466	7.0

Dinner:			
Huge Sunburst Salad		325	15.3
with Basic Dressing		150	trace
1 ear corn on the cob		70	2.0
1 cup steamed kale		45	5.0
	Total	590	22.3
	Daily Total	1190	35.5

THURSDAY

Breakfast:		Calories	Protein Grams
8 oz. fresh orange juice		110	2.0
12 pecan halves		81	1.1
	Total	191	3.1

Lunch:			
3 juicy ripe peaches		120	3.0
1 cup fresh strawberries		55	1.0
½ cup cottage cheese		117	14.0
	Total	292	18.0

Dinner:			
Huge Mixed Green Salad with Basic Dressing included		305	13.5
¼ recipe Whole-Wheat Linguine		335	7.0
1 cup steamed carrots		50	1.0
	Total	640	21.5
	Daily Total	1123	42.6

FRIDAY

Breakfast:		Calories	Protein Grams
8 oz. fresh Carrot and Celery Juice		142	12.1
½ ripe avocado		185	2.5
	Total	327	14.6

Lunch:			
Finger salad:			
3 small tomatoes		60	3.1
1 stalk celery		5	trace
1 small crisp cucumber		8	0.5
1 bowl of Hearty Black Bean Soup		300	15.0
	Total	373	18.6

Dinner:			
Large Mixed Green Salad, Tomato Dressing included		255	15.6
2 steamed potatoes in jackets with 2 pats butter		250	6.0
2 cups steamed cabbage		60	4.0
	Total	565	25.6
	Daily Total	1265	58.8

SATURDAY

Breakfast:		Calories	Protein Grams
Wedges of 1 whole pink grapefruit		100	2.0
½ cup cottage cheese		117	14.0
	Total	217	16.0

Lunch:			
1 ripe mango		120	1.0
3 peaches		120	3.0
6 soaked jumbo prunes		255	2.0
	Total	495	6.0

Dinner:			
large Buttercrunch Salad		110	9.0
with Basic Dressing		150	trace
2 rounds Eggplant Steak		350	15.0
1 cup steamed Swiss chard		27	2.7
	Total	637	26.7
	Daily Total	1349	48.7

SUNDAY

Breakfast:		*Calories*	*Protein Grams*
1 whole cantaloupe		160	4.0

Lunch:			
1 large bowl fresh Vegetable Soup		240	5.33
Super Sprouts salad		155	12.0
4 whole-wheat Venus wafers		72	2.0
	Total	**467**	**19.33**

Dinner:			
Huge Finger Salad, Basic Dressing included		278	5.6
2 baked potatoes, 1 pat butter each		360	4.0
1 cup steamed carrots		50	1.0
	Total	**688**	**10.6**

Snack:			
1 large pear		100	1.0
	Daily Total	**1415**	**34.93**

FOURTH WEEK

MONDAY

Breakfast:		*Calories*	*Protein Grams*
8 oz. fresh orange juice		110	2.0
½ cup natural pistachio nuts		297	9.5
	Total	**407**	**11.5**

Lunch:			
Green Goddess drink (15 minutes before the meal)		36	3.0
Pitacado		285	7.3
2 celery stalks		10	trace
	Total	**331**	**10.3**

Dinner:			
Large Born-Again Salad		80	15.0
1 whole baked acorn squash, 2 pats butter		200	4.0
1 cup steamed green peas		110	8.0
1 ear corn on the cob		70	2.0
	Total	**460**	**29.0**
	Daily Total	**1198**	**50.8**

TUESDAY

	Calories	Protein Grams
Breakfast:		
1 large slice ripe red watermelon	110	2.0
Lunch:		
½ recipe Fresh Fruit Special	264	10.2
Dinner:		
Large Spinach and Mushroom Salad, Basic		
Dressing included	262	18.5
1 cup Fresh Sweet Corn, Kentucky Style	137	2.3
1 cup steamed summer squash	30	2.0
Total	**429**	**22.8**
Snack:		
6 golden ripe apricots	110	2.0
Daily Total	**913**	**37.0**

WEDNESDAY

	Calories	Protein Grams
Breakfast:		
1 whole Spanish melon	240	2.8
Lunch:		
3 beefsteak tomatoes	99	4.8
2 large green celery stalks	10	trace
2 ounces natural Cheddar cheese	230	14.0
Total	**339**	**18.8**
Dinner:		
Texas-sized Sunburst Salad with ½ cup Avo-		
cado Dressing	433	18.3
1 cup steamed kale	45	5.0
1 baked potato, 1 pat butter	180	4.0
1 cup steamed cauliflower	30	3.0
Total	**688**	**30.3**
Daily Total	**1267**	**51.9**

THURSDAY

Breakfast:		Calories	Protein Grams
1 whole grapefruit		100	2.0
1 orange		65	1.0
¼ cup almonds		150	5.25
	Total	315	8.25

Lunch:		Calories	Protein Grams
½ recipe Fresh Fruit Special		264	10.2

Dinner:		Calories	Protein Grams
Buttercrunch Salad with Basic Dressing		260	9.0
1 baked yam, 1 pat butter		176	2.0
1 cup sliced beets		55	2.0
	Total	491	13.0
	Daily Total	1070	30.45

FRIDAY

Breakfast:		Calories	Protein Grams
3 ripe peaches		120	3.0
1 cup fresh raspberries		70	1.0
	Total	190	4.0

Lunch:		Calories	Protein Grams
1 cup of Vegetable Soup		120	2.66
1 Rica-dog		125	22.5
1 large stalk green celery		5	trace
	Total	250	25.16

Dinner:		Calories	Protein Grams
Mixed Vegetable Salad with Basic Dressing		269	21.0
½ recipe Squash à la Joy		148	2.4
1 cup Wild and Wonderful Rice, 1 pat butter		213	3.8
	Total	630	27.2

Snack:		Calories	Protein Grams
1 large banana		100	1.0
	Daily Total	1170	57.36

SATURDAY

Breakfast:		Calories	Protein Grams
½ fresh pineapple		140	0.5

Lunch:			
Mango Divine		245	4.4

Dinner:			
Finger Salad with ½ cup Avocado Dressing		236	8.6
1 small Baked Stuffed Eggplant		158	10.5
1 cup green steamed lima beans		170	10.0
1 cup steamed red cabbage		20	1.0
	Total	**584**	**30.1**

Snack:			
6 fresh figs		180	2.7
	Daily Total	**1149**	**37.7**

SUNDAY

Breakfast:		Calories	Protein Grams
1 papaya		156	2.4

Lunch:			
1 bowl Fresh Green Pea Soup		200	8.7
4 whole-wheat Venus wafers		72	2.0
2 celery stalks		10	trace
10 crisp green leaves romaine lettuce		17	1.7
	Total	**299**	**12.4**

Dinner:			
Mixed Green Salad, Basic Dressing included		305	13.5
1 cup Lentil Stew		180	10.0
Medium portion Broccoli Casserole		274	12.4
	Total	**659**	**35.9**

Snack:			
1 bunch of grapes		100	1.0
	Daily Total	**1214**	**51.7**

MONDAY

Breakfast:		Calories	Protein Grams
1 large wedge watermelon		110	2.0

Lunch:			
Finger Salad:			
3 ripe tomatoes		99	4.8
2 stalks crisp green celery		10	trace
1 small head Boston lettuce		25	2.0
2½ oz. Jarlsberg cheese		225	11.7
	Total	359	18.5

Dinner:			
Rainbow Salad with Basic Dressing		368	17.2
1 large baked potato, 2 pats butter		215	4.0
1 cup steamed beet greens		25	2.0
1 cup sliced beets		55	2.0
	Total	663	25.2

Snack:			
1 cup strawberries		55	1.0
	Daily Total	1187	46.7

TUESDAY

Breakfast:		Calories	Protein Grams
1 orange, sliced,		65	1.0
topped with ½ cup of			
blueberries and ¼ cup		45	0.5
grated fresh coconut		68.75	0.75
	Total	178.75	1.25

Lunch:			
2 cups steaming Creamy Corn Soup		230	5.0
4 rye thin wafers		90	4.0
1 whole cucumber, cut in strips		16	1.0
	Total	336	10.0

Dinner:			
Huge Rainbow Salad with Basic Dressing		368	17.2
1 baked potato, 1 pat butter		180	4.0
½ cup steamed green peas		55	4.0
	Total	603	25.2
	Daily Total	1182.75	37.45

Nibbling

Everyone gets the urge to nibble. The trick is to learn to handle the urge *rationally*. I make up Nibble Packs and keep them in the refrigerator. Before going to work, or off on a drive, or whatever, tuck a couple of Nibble Packs into your purse. They're *very* low in calories.

Nibble Pack #1. Into a small plastic sandwich bag put 10 two-inch celery pieces, 5 Kutter* cheese sticks.

Nibble Pack #2. 4 cherry tomatoes, one small pickle cucumber unskinned and cut into sticks. Bag.

Nibble Pack #3. 10 two-inch pieces of raw carrot, 10 small, cold, lightly steamed green beans. Bag.

Nibble Pack #4. 40 seedless white grapes. Bag.

Nibble Pack #5. 10 dark red bing cherries. Bag.

Nibble Pack #6. 2 cauliflower florets, 3 cherry tomatoes. Bag.

* Unsalted, unpasteurized cheese you can order by mail. Write the Kutter Cheese Co., Corfu, New York, for a price list.

BORN-AGAIN LIVING

CHAPTER 15

Exercise: Shape Up and Live Longer

In Africa, the fifteen- to fifty-year-old males of the Masai tribe walk twelve miles or more a day herding cattle. In studying the effects of this exercise on their hearts, Dr. George Mann of Vanderbilt University discovered something quite amazing. He divided the hearts into ten-year age groups and found that *the size of the coronary arteries increased with each decade of life.* The implication is inescapable that the exercise and fitness of the Masai cause their arteries to continue to grow throughout life rather than to become smaller, as is usually the case with sedentary, atherosclerosis-ridden individuals in America and other mechanized countries. The enlargement makes atherosclerosis or accumulation of sludge innocuous; the arteries are too large to become clogged.

Here's another way to look at exercise. In small but consistent doses it means permanent weight management, as long as it's continued indefinitely. By the time they've been out of school ten years, many Americans have gained thirty and even forty pounds of excess weight. One pound of fat equals 3500 stored calories which means that anyone who's forty pounds overweight has eaten and stored as fat 140,000 unneeded calories. For a 150-pound person, a brisk walk burns six or seven calories a minute. This means that had the individual put in less than ten minutes of walking per day over the ten-year period, he would never have gained those extra pounds!

REGULAR EXERCISE CAN BRING ABOUT BETTER CARDIOVASCU-
LAR EFFICIENCY, LOWER BLOOD PRESSURE, LOWER SERUM TRIGLY-
CERIDES, AND A BETTER RATIO OF HIGH-DENSITY TO LOW-DENSITY
LIPOPROTEINS. It probably increases coronary circulation and it
certainly promotes weight loss. All of these things promote
longevity.

THERE ARE FOUR KINDS OF EXERCISE, ALL HELPFUL IN DEVEL-
OPING ENDURANCE AS WELL AS SHAPING UP YOUR BODY. *Isotonics*
and *isometrics* involve the muscles. Isotonics exercise the muscles
through body movement, as in calisthenics or weight lifting. Isometrics involve no movement of the joints, only the muscles. You
can do valuable isometric exercise standing still, simply by con-
tracting and releasing a set of muscles, such as your pectorals.

Anaerobics and *Aerobics* bring oxygen to the body and exercise
heart and lungs by causing you to breathe deeply. Anaerobics do
this on a short-term basis. Walking, running, or bicycling for brief
distances provide anaerobic exercise.

Aerobics cause you to breathe deeply over a sustained period of
time, bringing oxygen to all your body's cells, where it combines
with glucose to provide energy. Of the four kinds of exercise, only
aerobics affects your entire system. Recently we've learned that
prolonged, strenuous exercise—extended bouts of running, jogging,
swimming, tennis, handball—are absolutely necessary, no matter
what your age, if you're going to look and feel terrific. A sluggish,
sedentary life leads to early aging, there's no longer any doubt
about it. Your whole system just slows down and clogs up, unless
you give it regular, strenuous exercise. To keep yourself pumping
along to a ripe and delicious old age, run like hell. Jump rope. Get
out there and play court games. MOVE! (Don't, however, leap up
from your office desk and begin to run the five miles home without
first learning how to build up your endurance. More on this later.)

I've done calisthenics just about every day of my life, from the
time I was fourteen years old. Now, at fifty, I follow a wonderfully
effective regimen that keeps every part of my body in great shape.
It's a regimen passed on to me by my cousin, Yvonne, a professional dancer. Yvonne returned to her career two years ago, at the
age of forty, after having taken time out while her children were
young. She needed a thorough, top-to-toe routine that was really
going to get her back in shape, and what she devised for herself
worked for me, so I'm going to pass it along to you. The exercises

are isotonics, and they do wonders. No jelly thighs or quivering un-derarms for those who keep up this routine. *But*—and this is a big but—isotonics, alone, won't really help you avoid premature aging. They don't exercise your heart sufficiently. So let me tell you a bit more about the aerobics program I've taken up. It's fun! I put on my running suit and running shoes, and then zip!, I'm out of the driveway and running down the road to a cul de sac that I use as my own private track. I trot around the track five, six, or as many times as I feel energetic enough to handle, back past the house, down the road another half a mile, and then back again through our field of buffalo grass to the swimming pool, where I take off my sweaty togs, grab a towel, and head for the water. After swimming four or five times the length of the pool, I jog back to the house to-tally refreshed and ready to take on the whole world.

These bouts of strenuous exercise have become so rewarding that I don't limit myself to working out once a day. Anytime I find ten minutes to spare, I slip out on the bicycle and hit the back road. When I've got the time I'll ride the three miles down the road to Pawling Health Manor and back.

So that I can't miss it as I go from the stairs to the kitchen, I keep a jump rope on the table in the foyer. It reminds me that I need even *more* exercise. Often I pick up the rope and start jump-ing. It takes less than a minute of vigorous jumping to get me breathing hard. The warm glow that takes over my body after this quick but good aerobic exercise is a good feeling—far better for starting the day than a hot cup of coffee.

LITERALLY, THE FIRE OF LIFE WILL BURN MORE EFFICIENTLY IN YOUR CELLS. Because this kind of exercise over a sustained period of time increases the supply of oxygen to your cells, it means that your entire metabolism is speeded up. Stored foodstuffs are broken down more efficiently and converted into living tissue. Waste mate-rial is more easily burned up and thrown out of your system. It's excreted in the sweat that pours out of you. Your blood circulates more vigorously to all parts of your body, including areas which have begun to deteriorate because of inactivity. Fat breaks down for use as fuel. Your heart beats faster. Your lungs work harder. You begin to feel warm all over. You begin to glow. You are liter-ally *more alive.*

If you've never done any serious running, bicycling, swimming, or other type of aerobic exercise, or haven't done it in a long time, begin cautiously. If you're over forty or have a history of heart or lung trouble, get an okay from your doctor before starting on a heavy walking or jogging program.

No matter who you are or what your age, it's a good idea to start slowly. Begin by walking and increase the length of your walk each day. Gradually walk faster, then jog short distances, walking between the jogging stints. After a week or two (depending upon age and physical condition) you'll probably be able to jog half a mile daily without difficulty. Gradually continue to increase your distance.

When I first began to jog, I did a half a mile a day. Now I'm jogging a mile a day and will increase the distance even more as I go along. In the first three weeks after I began jogging I lost an inch around my waist, noticed that my thighs had begun to firm up, and I was hooked!

If you live in a city apartment, you can jog around your block, as my cousin, Yvonne, does each morning. If you don't like that idea, you can run in place, in your own bedroom. When I began my aerobics program, I ran in my bedroom—six paces forward and six paces backward, keeping this up until I had a good breathing rhythm going.

Whatever your situation, if you really want to, you can include vigorous exercise in your daily routine. If you do, you may end up with changes in your life that are truly remarkable. A friend of mine, Dr. Donald Puretz, who's a member of the health education department at Dutchess Community College, in Poughkeepsie, N.Y., told me this amazing story.

Diary of a Long Distance Runner

"When I was thirty-five years old, in 1969, I signed up for some courses at the University of Rhode Island and noticed that there was a quarter-mile track on campus. While I considered myself to be in better physical condition than most American males my age—I played tennis and was still pitching in local baseball games—in fact, I was in horrendous shape. It's just that other men were in even worse shape, so I thought I was fine. In reality, while I didn't smoke or drink and got some exercise, I was at least twenty pounds overweight and had a blood-cholesterol level of 254 mg. per 100cc.

"The track was appealing. My first day on campus I thought

maybe I'd run a bit and thereby get myself in really ace condition. Having no idea where all this would eventually lead, I stripped to my blubbery self, put on shorts, tee shirt, and my trusty Converse sneakers, and sashayed over to the track. Once there, I began to jog very slowly, figuring I would just more or less take it easy until I was 'back in shape.' I did nine turns around the track—a total of two-and-a-quarter miles. My pulse rate, normally about 75, was up to 180.

"By the following morning my pulse was back in the mid-seventies and aside from a little stiffness, I felt okay. I decided to hit the track again. Days went by, weeks, and I continued to jog almost every day. Gradually my pulse rate became lower, my weight began to go down, and my blood pressure and cholesterol level dropped. By summer time I'd brought my weight down from 188 to 175—without dieting. My normal or resting pulse had become stabilized at about 60. My blood cholesterol was down to 175 and my blood pressure, which a year previously had been 135/85, was now 120/70. Without ever really deciding anything, I'd become a runner. My first two-and-a-quarter miles out on that track had taken twenty-three minutes and thirty seconds. Now I was running two miles in only thirteen minutes and fifty-five seconds. My mileage had also increased and I had begun taking long runs through the Dutchess County woods, which I think God made to order for jogging freaks.

"By 1972 I'd become a real runner. In that year alone I'd logged 800 miles! In three years of running my blood pressure had dropped to an amazing 100/60, I weighed a sleek 172, and still had not gone on a diet. I had run the mile in six minutes and five seconds flat, and could run an eight-minute mile for ten miles!

"In 1973, at the age of thirty-nine, I completed a fifteen-mile marathon in two hours, one minute and thirty-eight seconds. Today I'm still running, still hooked on this terrific sport, still maintaining my weight loss and low blood count and cholesterol level. Winter and summer, the trees fly past as I run. The sky is blue overhead. By running, as Eric Segal has said, I reaffirm my life!"

RUNNING HELPS NORMALIZE YOUR LUNGS, YOUR BLOOD PRESSURE, YOUR WEIGHT. While I'm not suggesting that you have to become a true long-distance runner, like Dr. Puretz, I wanted to share his story with you because I think it proves that getting outside and having a good run, on a regular basis, will make everything work better. Running will help you to feel, think and look better, and to live longer. *Never* get negative and think it's too late. Mr. E. E. Tutor, a retired merchant and farmer from Jackson, Mississippi, celebrated his eightieth birthday recently by jogging his daily, pre-dawn, two-mile route—a routine he started at the age of seventy-seven!

NOW I'D LIKE TO TELL YOU THE STORY OF MY COUSIN, YVONNE, WHOSE TERRIFIC PROGRAM OF BODY-SHAPING EXERCISES, WHICH I'M ABOUT TO SHARE WITH YOU, CAME OUT OF HER OWN BORN-AGAIN BODY EXPERIENCE. Yvonne grew up in the little town of Winchester, Kentucky. Her mother was my Aunt Fern, the sweet but misguided woman who plied me with all the sugary foods the summer I was fourteen and went to visit them. Yvonne was only three that summer. Because she is eleven years younger than I, we didn't really become friends until much later in life.

When Yvonne was in her teens, her family moved to Hollywood, California, and Yvonne eventually became a professional dancer. Because of her dancing she developed a beautiful, symmetrical body. But because of the eating habits she'd developed as a child and continued into adulthood, she had problems with acne, nerves, and poor digestion. Yvonne worked hard and fast. For breakfast she'd grab a couple of doughnuts and coffee. Lunch would be a hotdog washed down with a Coke or two. Dinner was often another fast, grab-what-you-can kind of meal.

In 1965, Yvonne went with a troupe to Korea to entertain American servicemen. During a performance she collapsed and had to be rushed to a hospital. Hemorrhaging ulcers. She was given immediate blood transfusions and later put on a bland diet.

Though she was hospitalized for over a week, it wasn't long before Yvonne began drifting back to her old food habits.

The following summer, in 1966, Yvonne came to New York to live. She telephoned me, and after not having seen each other for more than ten years, we became friends. At that time, Yvonne was a bit overweight and complained of stomach pains, now and again, though she continued to live on a diet that mainly consisted of spicy "fast" foods. She was also on lots of medication—hormones, tranquilizers, antacids.

When Yvonne made the trip up the Hudson to visit us for the first time, she was introduced to a way of life she'd never known. There were no medicines to be found in our house, no meat or processed foods of any kind. Yvonne listened as I explained why we ate the way we did, and why we believed in fasting. Soon she was on a three-day fast herself. (Because of emotional problems and her ulcer, it was all she could manage at the time.)

Gradually, Yvonne began to change many of her eating habits, and eventually became a vegetarian. In the years since then she's fasted a number of times. Slowly she was able to get off all the medication, including tranquilizers, on which she'd become dependent.

Yvonne met and married a wonderful man in New York, and soon had two children. The professional dancing stopped for a while and her muscles began to go soft. A few pounds crept back on the legs and thighs, where they were least wanted.

Last year, Yvonne decided it was time for a real shape-up. She put herself back onto a regular, daily exercise routine. On the following pages, she'll show you the simple exercises she still does to combat fat and flab in problem areas. Not unlike Shirley Mac-Laine, who, at age forty (after several sedentary years) had gained weight and lost her muscle tone, my wonderful dancer cousin put her will power to work and took out a new lease on life. As you'll see by the photographs in which she demonstrates her special body-shapers, Yvonne looks absolutely terrific. "You, too, can shape up, whether you're forty, fifty, or even sixty," says Yvonne. "All you need to do is *believe* that by putting in your time, religiously, your body will become wonderfully slim, firm, and flexible. Walking, running, and jumping will become pure joy."

Yvonne's Head-to-Toe Shape-up

Professional dancers know that in order for exercises to do what they're supposed to do, the body has to be relaxed and limber while it works out. The following routine incorporates relaxation or tension-reducing exercises, which you'll do along with the special, body-shaping exercises through which you'll overcome particular figure problems. Just follow Yvonne, from top to toe, from Exercise 1, a simple head roll, to Exercise 20, a simple ankle circle. It's a gentle enough routine that you can start right out with, going straight through from Exercise 1 to 20. *Relax, take your time, and never, never push or strain yourself.* As the days pass, and you find yourself getting stronger and more limber, you can *increase the repetitions* of the exercises, devoting special attention to those areas of your body that need it.

Exercise 1: The Head Roll

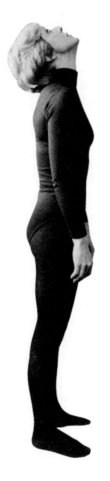

With your body relaxed, knees straight and feet apart, let your head drop forward. Slowly roll head back as far as you're able while at the same time jutting your chin forward. Repeat.

Drop chin toward chest. Then, with head, describe a large circle, rolling head first toward right shoulder, then back, then to left shoulder and front again. Then raise chin, drop head forward again, and repeat, going from left to right this time.

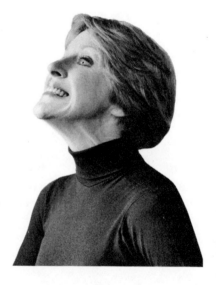

Exercise 2: The Face and Neck Relaxer

With teeth clamped together, smile as wide as you can. Hold a beat. Relax. Repeat. (Simple? And how good it makes your face feel after a while.)

Exercise 3: The Shoulder Tuck
(FOR GETTING LOOSE)

Standing relaxed, with feet slightly apart, tuck shoulder up under earlobes by pulling up hard, then dropping it down. Repeat.

Alternate one shoulder at a time. Then do both.

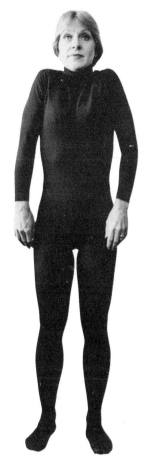

Exercise 4: Shoulder Circles
(FOR GETTING LOOSE)

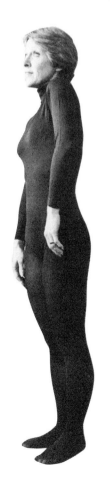

With the idea of describing a large circle with your shoulders, pull *just* your shoulders forward, then (smoothly) up under the earlobes, then back, then down. Do both shoulders together.

Alternate, doing a right shoulder circle, then a left shoulder circle. Reverse. Concentrate on staying loose.

Exercise 5: Arm Circle Swing
(FOR BEGINNING TO FLY)

Hold both arms in front of you at bust height, keeping elbows straight and letting your fingertips touch. Keeping arms at same height, swing them behind you, touching fingertips again behind your back. Repeat, swinging arms backward, then forward, backward, then forward, building a nice, loose rhythm. (Whee! Feel the energy start to build?)

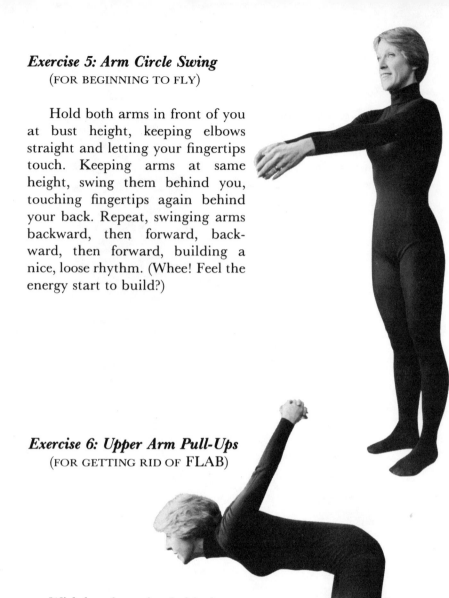

Exercise 6: Upper Arm Pull-Ups
(FOR GETTING RID OF FLAB)

With hands resting behind you, on buttocks, interlock fingers. Keeping elbows straight, pull your shoulders back (hands still clasped). Now, with hands still clasped, raise arms up behind you as far as you can (up, up, up) while bending over from the waist.

Stand up and relax, with arms at sides. Repeat.

Exercise 7: Elbow Circles
(LOOSENING UP AND SHAPING UP)

Rest hands lightly on shoulders, holding elbows forward at shoulder height. Using elbows to describe a circle, smoothly roll elbows up, then back behind you, then down at sides, then forward. Repeat 5 times.

Roll elbows in reverse, 5 times. Elbows to the back, then down, then up, then forward.

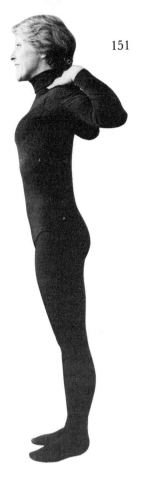

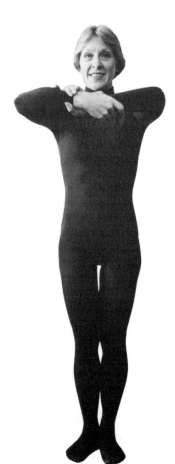

Exercise 8: Bust Shape-up
(THIS IS GOOD FOR EVERYONE, SMALL, MEDIUM, OR LARGE.

IT'S FOR FIRMNESS AND SHAPE.)

Standing relaxed, with feet slightly apart, hold arms in front of you with elbows bent. Grasp right wrist with left hand and left wrist with right hand. With sharp, rhythmic motions (one-two-three-four) push wrists toward elbows. (No mystery about *this* exercise. You can feel what's happening immediately.)

Exercise 9: Swinging Waist-Whittler

Sitting tailor-fashion on the floor, raise your arms up in front of you with elbows at shoulder height. Bend your arms at the elbow, with middle fingertips touching, and swing arms as far as they'll go to the right, then to the left. Repeat.

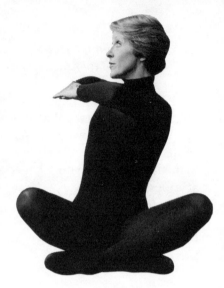

Exercise 10: Sit-Ups

(TO MAKE YOUR ABDOMEN AS FIRM AND FLAT AS CHER'S, WHOSE COSTUME DESIGNER SAYS SHE HAS "THE BEST BELLY IN HOLLYWOOD.")

TRADITIONAL VERSION

Lie flat on your back, on the floor, and put your arms straight up alongside your head. With your legs kept flat against the floor and your knees kept straight and toes pointed, pull your torso up in a sitting position. That's right, pull, pull, pull—you're up! Remember to keep your spine straight while doing this one. (Didn't you feel the pull on your belly? A few months of this and Cher will have nothing on you.)

BEGINNER'S VERSION
(VERY EFFECTIVE, SO DON'T UNDER-ESTIMATE)

Tuck your toes under a couch, a low chair, or another piece of heavy furniture to stabilize yourself. Lie flat on your back with hands clasped behind head and knees slightly bent. Do your sit-ups as above—6 or 8 of them to start.

Exercise 11: Waist Rolls

(FOR WAIST AND STOMACH)

Bend forward at the waist with your arms hanging down, relaxed. Keeping your feet planted firmly and slightly apart, slowly roll to the right as far as you can go. Roll backward, with stomach protruding in a relaxed way; continue rolling left, then forward. Do twice, then reverse.

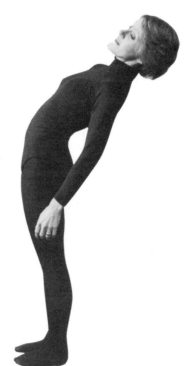

Exercise 12: The Bump

(DYNAMITE FOR HIPS—AND FUN! DO THIS WITH MUSIC, IF YOU LIKE.)

Stand with feet apart, knees slightly bent, and arms at sides. Keeping torso faced straight ahead and perfectly still, thrust pelvis forward in a sharp bump, belly-dancer style. Just as sharply, thrust buttocks backward. Go from back to front 8 times.

Again, keeping torso stationary, thrust right hip to side with a sharp bump. Repeat on left side.

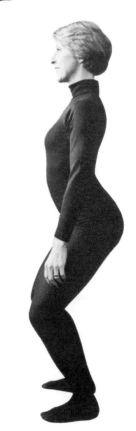

Exercise 13: Circle Bump

(GOOD FOR BUTTOCKS, WAIST, ABDOMEN)

Take the two types of Bump you learned in Exercise 12, put it all together in the form of a circle. Stand with feet apart, knees slightly bent, and arms hanging loose at sides. Facing front, with torso held stationary, bump your pelvis first to the right, and back to center. Then thrust backward and forward. Then thrust left, and back. Then thrust forward, and back.

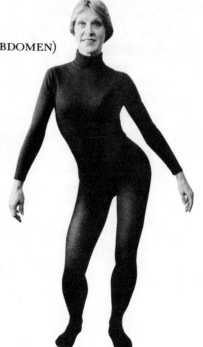

Exercise 14: The Thigh Thinner

(BE SURE TO DO THIS ONE IN FRONT OF A MIRROR)

With feet planted firmly and slightly apart on the floor, bend your left leg. With your torso bent slightly forward for balance, pick up your right ankle and place on your left knee. Raise right arm above your head, and then reach forward with it, pulling forward with your upper torso. (Feel the stretch, stretch, stretch.) Slowly lower right arm to bust height. You should now be in a semi-sitting position, with buttocks tucked in nicely. Maintain your forward-reaching stance. Now, while pushing your right knee toward the floor and pointing your right toe, keep stretching forward to the count of 5.

Repeat on other side.

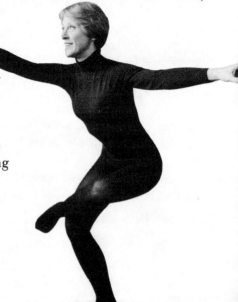

Exercise 15: Thigh-Thinner Roll

Sit on the floor with back straight and soles of feet together, hands clasped around toes. Roll sideways to the right, touching right knee to floor. Roll sideways to the left, touching left knee to floor. Rock and roll, right and left, building a relaxed rhythm.

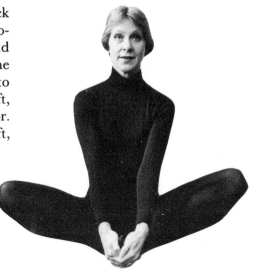

Exercise 16: Wall Push-Up
(FOR FIRM, SHAPELY CALVES)

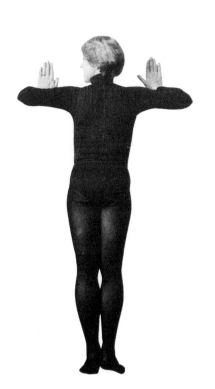

Stand with knees straight and feet slightly apart, facing a wall. Keeping elbows straight, place hands in front of you, palms flat against the wall, at shoulder height. Keeping palms on wall, walk backward as far as you can and still be comfortable while flat-footed.

Keeping feet firmly planted, heels down, lean forward and touch right cheek to wall. Straighten elbows. Then lean forward again with elbows bent and touch other cheek to wall. Do this exercise up to 6 times.

Exercise 17: Inner-Thigh Stretch
(FOR GETTING RID OF THOSE RIPPLES)

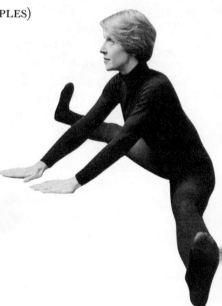

Sitting on the floor with back straight, spread legs as far apart as possible, keeping knees straight and toes turned up. Place hands palm-down on the floor, directly in front of your pelvis. Walk hands slowly forward, and you'll feel the ligaments of your inner thighs stretch. Slowly lower your elbows to the floor and place full weight on forearms. Gently lean into this position and hold until the stretch begins to hurt good. Straighten up slowly and bring legs together S-L-O-W-L-Y.

Exercise 18: Leg Lifts
(THESE SHAPE UP THE WHOLE LEG NICELY)

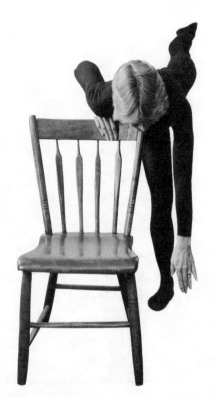

Place your right hand on the back of a sturdy chair. Lean forward and lift your left leg behind you, keeping your knee straight and toes pointed. Keep leaning forward and lifting your leg as far as you can. Work toward touching the floor with your left finger tips and bouncing the extended leg gently, 5 or 6 times.

Reverse, and lift the right leg.

Exercise 19: Foot Flexer

(NEVER OVERLOOK YOUR FEET; YOU CAN GET MORE TOTAL RE-
LAXATION FASTER FROM EXERCISING YOUR FEET THAN ANY OTHER
PART OF YOUR BODY.)

Sit on the floor with your back straight, your legs straight in front of you and knees together, with palms flat on the floor at your sides.

First, point toes forward. Then flex toes up and turn feet out while keeping toes flexed. Close feet together (toes still flexed). Repeat this foot routine rhythmically, to the count of four. Repeat.

Exercise 20: Ankle Circles

(TO COMPLETE YOUR BODY WORKOUT)

Sitting in the same position as for the previous exercise, lift your right heel about six inches off the floor. Concentrate on relaxing the foot, and draw circles in the air with your right big toe. Repeat with left foot.

YVONNE USES EXERCISE TO COMBAT STRESS. She has two lovely fantasy exercises which I'm going to share with you. Ideally, you should do them every day to keep stress from getting the upper hand, but you can also do them after the fact, when stress has already taken its toll on you.

THE MAGICAL LIQUID. Lie in bed (you should try to do this even before getting up in the morning), close your eyes, and concentrate on your body. Visualize each part of it—heart, lungs, arms, legs, brain—and imagine that each part is connected to a tube filled with soothing, refreshing liquid. In your mind's eye, observe this liquid passing slowly throughout your system, section by section. The liquid is removing all negatives and replacing them with positives. It's invigorating every single cell in your body. Imagine that you can see the liquid as it flows. Mentally direct the liquid to flow to any part of your body that especially needs it. If you lie quietly and tune in to every part of yourself, if you *listen*, you'll be able to identify the parts of your body that are really feeling the stress, and with that "liquid" energy, you can heal them.

THE BELLOWS OF LIFE. Think of your diaphragm as if it were an accordion. The air you take into your "bellows" becomes life-force as you blow the air out. You can take a few of these special breaths whenever you're feeling hectic or pressured. Just let the air in, all the way down to your diaphragm, and let the diaphragm push it out again, as fresh, new energy for you.

CHAPTER 16

The Breath of Life

AN ADEQUATE SUPPLY OF GOOD, UNPOLLUTED OXYGEN AND PROPER BREATHING ARE AS ESSENTIAL TO NUTRITION AS EATING THE RIGHT FOOD.

Remember the four functions the cells must perform in order for you to be nourished:

1) They must break down or digest food.
2) They must assimilate nutrients.
3) They must respire, or take in oxygen.
4) They must excrete, or let off carbon dioxide.

The last two processes, respiration and excretion, are as vital as the first two.

RESPIRATION GOES HAND IN HAND WITH CIRCULATION.

Let's examine these two processes to see what they do for us. Both can be expedited! Both can contribute to the Born-Again Body!

When you breathe, you are drawing air into the lungs by the action of the diaphragm, a muscle somewhat like a piece of rubber sheeting that stretches across the chest, separating the chest cavity from the abdomen. Like the heart's, the action of the diaphragm is usually automatic, but we actually can learn to operate it better, *consciously,* and step up the supply of oxygen! (I will give some special exercises for this later in the chapter.)

When the diaphragm expands (or when we consciously expand

it), the size of the chest cavity is increased. This creates a vacuum and fresh air rushes in to fill it. When the diaphragm relaxes, it rises up, making the chest and lungs contract, and we exhale.

The fresh oxygen we get when we inhale must make contact with the blood, in the lungs. Here's how it happens.

Bright red and laden with nutrients, blood is pumped through the arteries to every part of the body, where it nourishes the cells. The used blood then returns to the heart via the veins. Burdened with wastes, the used blood (now dull and blue) goes to the right ventricle of the heart, which pumps it on into the lungs. There it's distributed by millions of hairlike blood vessels to the air cells that line the lungs.

A MIRACULOUS SWITCH-OFF TAKES PLACE IN THE LUNGS. When you inhale, you bring fresh oxygen into contact with your old, used blood. It happens through the thin walls of those hairlike blood vessels. The walls of these vessels are thick enough to contain the blood, but thin enough to allow precious oxygen to penetrate them. When the oxygen contacts the blood, a miraculous switch-off occurs. The blood takes up the good, fresh oxygen, and at the same time gets rid of the carbon dioxide gas, CO_2, generated from the toxins and waste matter that have been gathered by the blood from all parts of the body. Thus purified and oxygenated, the blood is then ready to make another life-giving trip through the body.

The *way* you breathe makes all the difference.

Considering how important oxygen is to the human metabolism, the manner in which you breathe is vital. (Earlier, primitive forms of humans undoubtedly breathed right naturally, but civilization, which has made us tense and rigid, has also affected our natural breathing.)

SHALLOW BREATHING IS IMPERFECT BREATHING. It brings only a portion of the lung cells into play, which means the body is then *under*-oxygenated. From the standpoint of proper physiological functioning, then, the techniques of breathing hold the promise of better health. (Some think they also hold the promise of a kind of sensuous pleasure unknown to those for whom breathing remains unconscious. I happen to agree with them.)

In his book, *Meta-calisthenics,* Lowell G. Miller describes two *wrong* kinds of breathing and two *right* kinds. The wrong kinds, he says, are the "high" or "shoulder" breathing—raising your shoulders and breathing up high, at the base of the throat—and the very common "middle" breathing—expanding your chest by pushing out your ribs. The latter is actually a caricature of proper breathing (picture the army sergeant swelling out his chest for inspection). In fact, when you swell out your chest to breathe—and do only that—you end up using only about half your lungs' capacity.

THE TWO RIGHT WAYS TO BREATHE ARE THE "DEEP BREATH" AND THE "COMPLETE BREATH." The deep breath must be learned before you can do the complete breath. To do the deep breath you are going to put into action your diaphragm—that muscle that covers the abdomen in an arc and protrudes up into the chest cavity like a hill. You will consciously use your diaphragm to push your abdomen *down* and out of the way, thus creating a space in the lung cavity for the lungs to *expand*.

The lower lungs are allowed to fill only when the diaphragm is expanded. This is the only way air can enter the important depths of the lungs. In deep or "low" breathing, your stomach will appear to swell *down* and *out*. Though deep (or low, or abdominal) breathing is vastly better than middle and high breathing, in terms of total air and oxygen intake, it is still no match for the complete breath. This is a super type of breathing practiced by Eastern yogis which Western health buffs have discovered is like a little "cure" all its own.

THE COMPLETE BREATH WILL RAISE THE OXYGEN LEVEL OF YOUR BLOOD TO A SUPER ENERGETIC HIGH. It also aids in the expulsion of toxins and wastes. It is such a vigorous form of breathing that it actually kneads or massages the inner organs. Instructions for the complete breath are:

1) Stand or sit erect, to allow for free expansion of the lungs. Then inhale steadily through the nostrils, filling the lower lungs (as in the deep breath) by distending the diaphragm. (Your stomach should swell from the groin up.)

2) Smoothly, without jerking, fill the middle of the lungs by pushing out first the lower ribs, next the lower chest. (See illustration.) Only then, fill the high space by protruding your chest and raising your shoulders. Retain this big breath as long as you can.

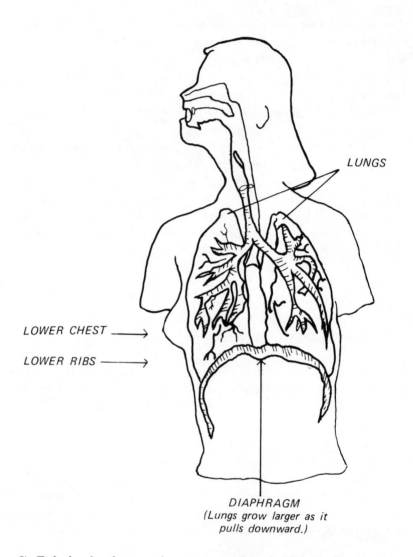

LUNGS

LOWER CHEST ——→

LOWER RIBS ——→

DIAPHRAGM
*(Lungs grow larger as it
pulls downward.)*

3) Exhale slowly, not in a great whoosh. Gradually contract and raise the abdomen, then the middle area, then the high area. After practice, you should be able to exhale so quietly you don't hear the air coming out. But do exhale fully! Remember, you're getting rid of toxins. To squeeze out all the "bad" air, let your chest and diaphragm collapse a bit.

If you think all this sounds elaborate, it isn't. It's the way nature intended us to breathe. The next time you see an infant who hasn't been made tense and anxious by the world he lives in, watch the way he breathes.

The deep breath and the complete breath are the basics. Practice them until they're second nature. Special breathing exercises for instant energy, for relaxation and rest, and for restoring natural lung space are included in "30 Days to a New You," the special living regimen at the end of this book.

Why Breathing Properly Is Essential

To build a good fire in your fireplace you need excellent dry wood, paper, and matches to start the fire. If you don't arrange the logs so that oxygen can reach them easily, they will smolder rather than burn. By the same token, if you let too many ashes accumulate, the fire will smother. Having fine, dry wood isn't sufficient in and of itself; you must also have a ready supply of oxygen.

Getting oxygen to your cells and getting rid of their waste material is as important to your life as supplying oxygen to the wood in your fireplace and emptying the ashes.

OXYGEN COMBINES WITH FUEL (GLUCOSE) IN YOUR BLOODSTREAM TO FORM ENERGY. The heat that's generated by the combustion of oxygen and glucose in your cells provides heat for the maintenance of normal body temperature. It also generates energy for breathing, walking, thinking, and every other physical and mental activity. *Without sufficient oxygen, all these functions become impaired.*

Anything you do that interferes with your body's processes of oxygenation and the removal of carbon dioxide causes your cells slowly to become exhausted. Eventually they could even starve to death. Two things happen:

» Your cells become saturated with their own wastes. (This is like forcing them to exist in a sewer polluted by their own excretions.)
» They are unable to generate the heat needed to provide you with energy. When you exert yourself playing tennis, say, or even climbing the stairs—activities you should be able to perform effortlessly—you find yourself becoming short of breath. Your extremities may also get cold.

What sorts of interference create these problems? Breathing stale or polluted air, for starters. Also smoking, being overweight, and being physically inactive.

Breathing stale air actually forces you to take back into your lungs waste substances that have already been excreted, either from yours or other people's cells. When your breath smells bad, it's simply the excreta, in gas form, from your cells' waste materials. (Unless, of course, the odor's caused by unhealthy teeth and gums.) When you stay in a closed room with no fresh air circulating, what you're doing is taking that excreta back into your system.

POLLUTION KILLS. When you breathe polluted air, you take poisonous chemicals into your bloodstream. They upset the oxygen balance by robbing your cells of valuable space. Aside from the cancer-triggering results of ingesting such chemicals as nicotine, benzopyrine, betanepthylamine, methancholanthrine, carbon monoxide, hydrocarbons, phenols, aldehydes, and cyanide (to name just a few), their oxygen-depriving effects alone are devastating to your health.

CIGARETTE SMOKE: THE BREATH OF DEATH. If you inhale a pack of cigarettes a day you're ingesting a cup of tar a year into your lungs. This accumulation paralyzes their defenses. Your lungs form extra mucus in order to trap foreign materials. Soon the cilia, the little hairlike structures lining your lungs, are unable to get rid of the mucus because they've been weighted down by the tar. The macrophages, or suction cells, that rid the lungs of harmful substances, slowly become inactive.

Smoking drastically impairs your lungs' ability to take in oxygen and get rid of carbon dioxide. The impairment is slow death to your cells. Based on statistics arrived at by Dr. Raymond Pearl of Johns Hopkins University, Andrew Salter, in his book, *Conditioned Reflex Therapy,* stated: "The heavy smoker pays with 34.6 minutes of his life for each cigarette he smokes. The pack-a-day smoker pays with 11.5 hours for each pack he smokes."

When you smoke you're laying the groundwork for your own premature death. If you're still smoking, regardless of all the evidence that's been presented to you over the last ten years, why not ask yourself the following questions.

» Do you value yourself enough to want to live your life out to its fullest?

» Do you care about making as many of your own small contributions to humankind as possible?

» Do you want to deprive your children and other loved ones at a time in their lives when they may need you most?

Just as smoking interferes seriously with the processes that must be carried out by your lungs, so does fat. Your lungs weren't designed to supply oxygen to a body encumbered by fat.

BEING OVERWEIGHT INTERFERES WITH NORMAL BREATHING. Your lungs aren't able to increase in size to match the rest of you. All they can do is struggle along trying to get the necessary oxygen to all the extra fat cells you've manufactured.

When you have an accumulation of fat hanging around your abdomen it restricts your breathing. Not only that, the air sacs in your lungs become infiltrated with fat, cutting down on the volume of air your lungs can handle. Put an overweight or obese person in a race with a person of normal weight and see who begins to pant for breath and fall by the wayside first!

EXERCISE IS VITAL FOR DEVELOPING HIGH-POWERED RESPIRATION. Think about it. Your body was designed to perform vigorous, sustained exercise—like running, bicycling, swimming—which makes you breathe deep and hard over a sustained period of time. The heart beats faster than normal and eventually becomes stronger. The oxygen capacity of your lungs increases. Oxygen travels more easily to all the cells and tissues in your body, which increases your overall health and energy level. Activity is taking place in your cells! Stored fat is being used up. Your muscle tissue becomes harder. All your tissues become firmer and healthier. Without oxygen, these miraculous changes couldn't take place.

SIX THINGS YOU CAN DO TO HELP YOURSELF TO THE BREATH OF LIFE.

1) Live and work in well-ventilated rooms. Keep fresh air circulating in the rooms you occupy. If you use a woodburning stove in the winter, be aware that it burns up oxygen, which must be replenished.

Spend as much time outdoors as you can. If you live in the city, try to get into the country as often as possible.

2) Avoid, to the degree that you're able, heavily trafficked

areas, industrial areas, and smoke-filled rooms. As a non-smoker, demand your rights.

3) If you smoke, give it up. It's deadly, that's all.

4) Exercise, exercise, exercise.

5) Eat an abundance of raw, green leafy vegetables and other foods that contain chlorophyl. Chlorophyl helps make healthy red blood cells, and the more of those you have, the more efficiently your respiratory processes can function.

6) If you're overweight, *lose!* You can begin by following the regimen in Chapter 7, "Fasting to Look Younger (and Lose Weight)." Follow that by reading the chapter, "A New Solution for the Overweight."

Breath is life. Determine *now* to add both quality and quantity to your life by improving your breath!

CHAPTER 17

Sun:
the Super Energizer

Do you know why being in the sun makes you feel so good?

» Sunshine stimulates the pituitary gland, which, in turn, stimulates the production of melanin-related hormones called melanocytes. The more of those hormones we have, the greater our sense of well-being.

» Sun also tends to lower blood pressure, possibly accounting for the fact that so many people fall asleep at the beach.

» Research with animals has shown the effects of sun on the pineal gland, which has a stimulating effect on certain sex hormones. It's been proved that there's a direct correlation between the mating of birds, for example, and the amount of sunshine present.

» Sunshine is known to be psychically restorative, one of nature's anti-depressants, which may be why Latins, as well as races close to the equator, are known for being fun-loving, while the Nordic people have the highest suicide rate—especially during winter, when there is no sun at all!

The sun is the source of energy for all plants, and, indirectly, for all animals. The energy produced when you burn coal or wood or gasoline or oil is exactly the same energy that enables you to move, talk, breathe, and think.

» The heat and energy that's produced by fire comes from the sun's energy that was stored in the tree which eventually ended up as firewood.

» The energy produced by burning coal comes from the sun's energy that was stored in the ferns and green plants which over millions of years decomposed and became coal.

» The petroleum pumped from the depths of the earth was once tiny plants whose stored sun energy is released when it's combusted in the engine of your car.

PLANTS HAVE THE ABILITY TO TRAP AND STORE SUN ENERGY. The heat and energy released by oxidation in your cells comes from the plant food you eat, either directly, or when you eat animals that have fed on plants.

Only plants can trap the sun's energy and store it for later use. All animals are dependent on plants to supply them with the precious, life-giving fuel. Without the sun-energy you get from plants, you wouldn't be able to live.

PLANTS PRODUCE THEIR OWN FOOD AND ENERGY BY A PROCESS CALLED PHOTOSYNTHESIS. Four things are required for photosynthesis: carbon dioxide, light, water, and chlorophyl. The plant gets the carbon dioxide it needs from the air, which enters the leaves through little openings called stomata. Water is obtained from the soil.

With the aid of chlorophyl (the green coloring matter in the plant) and the radiant energy provided by sunlight, the raw materials—carbon dioxide and water—are changed into sugar, which is stored by the plant and used when needed. Some of the unused sugar is changed into starch and fat and stored for future use. Some is changed into proteins and vitamins.

During photosynthesis oxygen is formed. Some of it is used by the plant to burn its food and release energy.

YOU GET YOUR ENERGY FROM EATING THE PLANT. In fact, when you depend on other animals rather than plants for your energy, you're getting it in diluted form. By the time you sink your teeth into a steak, most of the cow's stored sun-energy has already been used by the cow. Meat-eating is an inefficient way to get your sun power!

Green leaves are the powerhouses of vitamins, minerals, distilled water, and amino acids, the building blocks of protein. When you eat green leafy vegetables you're literally eating stored sun power. Vegetables provide the most efficient supply of building materials (or protein) your body can use and fruit provides the most efficient supply of energy (sugar) your body can use.

DIRECT CONTACT WTH THE SUN'S RAYS IS NECESSARY FOR THE PRODUCTION OF VITAMIN D. Certain of the sun's life-giving rays you must get directly for yourself; the plant can't do it for you. This is true of the ultraviolet rays. Ultraviolet is a catalyst for the formation of Vitamin D in your system. It also helps you make use of calcium and phosphorous that's in the food you eat.

WHAT HAPPENS WHEN WE DON'T GET SUNLIGHT?

Cover a patch of your beautiful green lawn with a piece of canvas or any other opaque material. In a matter of days the grass underneath will turn white and die.

Enclose a sturdy tomato plant in a colored glass container. Watch the tomatoes grow large inside but never ripen.

Feed two puppies the same diet but keep one in a dark closet and allow the other to spend its days out in the sunshine. The dog that's kept in the closet will be weak, stunted, and short-lived.

YOU CAN VASTLY INCREASE YOUR HEALTH AND ENERGY POTENTIAL THROUGH PROPER USE OF THE SUN.

I have found the sun to be an essential ingredient in my quest for healthy skin. There's no doubt that it's been a healing force in the management of my psoriasis.

You, too, can improve your health and greatly increase your zest for life through careful use of the sun. Here are some suggestions to help you do just that.

1) Let the sunlight into your home. Keep the shades up, the blinds open, and let your color schemes be light ones that reflect rather than subdue sunlight. It's been proved that a lack of sunlight actually contributes to depression.

2) If you're a student, study in natural daylight whenever you can. Scientific studies show that you learn better in natural light than you do in artificial.

3) Every day that you can, take a sunbath exposing as much of your body as possible. If you have a private sunning spot, sunbathe nude. But *do* exercise caution and good sense, as excessive exposure to the strongest rays of the sun has been known to trigger skin cancer in people with certain types of skin.

» Especially if you're over thirty-five, prolonged sunbathing should stop at about 11 A.M. and not start again until 3 P.M. The higher the sun in the sky, the more burning its ultraviolet rays.

- » If you are a natural blond or redhead you should exercise special caution, especially when you first start sunning in the summer.
- » If you haven't been exposed to the sun for several weeks or months, your first sunning sessions should be short—ten or fifteen minutes the first day, and gradually increasing the period of exposure. *How* gradually depends upon how prone to burning you are.
- » Remember that sunshine and certain kinds of drugs don't mix. *The Pill* causes ultrasensitivity to sun—and "sun spots" on the skin—in some individuals.
- » When compounded by the natural, tranquilizing effects of the sun, *tranquilizers* can cause adverse reactions. *Diuretics* may prove *more* dangerous in the sun because they plunge your blood pressure and the sun already lowers blood pressure to some extent. Even aspirin behaves strangely in the sun. For one thing, it tends to (temporarily) eliminate redness in pigmentation, so that if you take aspirin before sunbathing it could obscure any clue as to how much sunburn you're getting.

If you live in a cold or temperate climate and can afford to travel south in the winter, you'll find that a trip to warm, sunny climes—Florida, the Caribbean islands, Palm Springs, Hawaii—will restore your lagging levels of Vitamin D and quickly renew your spirits and energy level.

If you're unable to get away, you'd be surprised at how much you can accomplish for yourself in a sheltered, sunny corner or on a flat, protected rooftop. The winter I was eighteen my psoriasis flared up. I was determined to get some sun, which I knew would help to control the problem. I found a sheltered spot on the roof covering the front porch. It was quite handy as I could climb right out onto it from my bedroom window. Each day I'd spend some time when the sun was at its highest lying on my rooftop and looking down at the snow covering the ground below. (This was in the mountains of North Carolina.) By early March my skin was so smooth and tan that a friend asked, "Have you been to Florida?"

Sunbathing is considered a luxury (or an indulgence) by many, but it shouldn't be. We desperately need the sun's rays to counteract the indoor lives we lead. Remember, humans weren't designed to spend forty or fifty hours a week indoors, doing close work under the buzz of fluorescent lighting. So make the time for yourself, and find your own little "place in the sun." You'll soon begin to look better and feel better. You'll soon be saying, "This is wonderful! Why didn't I ever do this before?"

CHAPTER 18

Four Kinds of Rest
for Health and Beauty

Few of us are truly relaxed, serene, and fully rested. We tend to be a people who work past the point of natural fatigue, who give ourselves artificial stimulants in order to keep going, and who then drug ourselves with liquor or sleeping pills to be able to relax enough to get to sleep.

Chances are you don't understand how profoundly your body needs adequate rest. Dr. Hans Selye, the scientist who discovered the importance of stress as a disease factor in modern life, wrote:

> *Many people believe that after they have exposed themselves to very stressful activities, a rest can restore them to where they were before. This is false.*

"Experiments on animals," Dr. Selye went on to say, "have clearly shown that each exposure leaves an indelible scar, in that it uses up reserves of adaptability which cannot be replaced."

While it's true that after a highly stressful experience or activity a good rest can restore almost all of your original vigor, the state of your total organism will never be quite what it was before. "Just a little deficit of adaptation energy every day adds up," Selye observed. What it adds up to is aging.

We use up energy just by the fact of living. Any expenditure of energy as you work, play, eat, think, make love, drive, jog, swim— even sleep—lowers, to some extent, your reserves of energy. It also causes wear and tear on the organism. Living itself is in part a "using up" process.

THIS BREAKING DOWN AND USING UP IS THE PROCESS OF "CATABOLISM."

»　De-amination or the breaking down of complicated proteins into their basic amino acids is an example of a catabolic process.

»　The mechanism whereby harmful chemical additives are sorted out of the digested food and either excreted or stored away is another example.

THE BODY HAS A COMPENSATORY BUILDING UP PROCESS CALLED "ANABOLISM."

During rest and sleep your cells do an entirely different kind of work. They speed up waste removal. They also speed up the processes of repair and renewal.

»　During sleep, high levels of growth hormone are produced. This stimulates tissue growth, speeds healing, and lowers blood cholesterol—all anabolic processes.

»　The useful enzymes and hemoglobin created as a result of amino acid breakdown constitute another anabolic process.

THE CLOSELY RELATED PROCESSES OF ANABOLISM AND CATABOLISM ARE CALLED "METABOLISM."

For your body to operate smoothly and for you to be in good health, there must be a high degree of balance between the tearing down and the building up processes within your cells, tissues, and organs. Metabolic efficiency determines your basic energy level. When you take in more unusable material—junk food, chemicals, saturated fats, and even protein—than your system can handle, and when you don't get enough compensatory rest, your metabolism goes out of whack and your body gradually enters a state of dis-ease.

THE HEALTHY BODY REQUIRES FOUR DIFFERENT KINDS OF REST. Sometimes you can refresh yourself with just one or two, but periodically—6 to 8 hours out of every day—your system demands all four.

Physical Rest is obtained by ceasing motor activity and relaxing. You can get a certain amount of rest just sitting, though it's more restful to lie down. It's most restful of all to sleep.

Mental Rest occurs when your mind is free from worry, and—to the degree that it's possible—thought. Mental activity uses up a terrific amount of energy, whether it's the energy used in problem solving or the energy used *avoiding* problem solving. Have you ever been worried or uptight about something, only to find that when you lie down to rest, you can't? Your body is lying perfectly still but your mind is racing? A complete rest must include the mental as well as physical.

Sensory Rest is being able to "float free" for awhile and rest those nerve endings that are responsible for your sensory perceptions. To achieve sensory rest you have to be in a place where you can block out noise, smells, tastes, sights, and all tactile sensations, concentrating on nothing but the sweet rise and fall of your own diaphragm as you breathe.

Physiological Rest involves your internal organs. When you stop eating and fast, you are giving a physiological rest to your digestive system. Fasting lifts the workload from the digestive organs and allows that energy to be used instead by the processes of elimination and repair. It's like shifting gears. Your system goes into a completely different operation: that of excreting the waste material from cells.

As you learned in Chapter 16, cellular excretion goes on continuously. However, when you fast, thereby freeing the energy used by digestion for use in elimination, the process of excreting toxins and wastes from your system is definitely accelerated. The end result is a very special kind of rest for your body. This rest lays the groundwork for more efficient renewal and repair.

ALL FOUR KINDS OF REST OCCUR WHEN YOU SLEEP. The process of repair and renewal in your body is best accomplished during the sleep state. During sleep your mental activities are reduced; your digestive system is at rest; your senses are at rest, and your physical self is at its most relaxed. Without this daily period of complete rest your total organism would begin to break down.

DRUG-INDUCED SLEEP DEPLETES YOUR VITALITY. Artificially induced sleep is deficient in comparison with natural sleep. It's destructive to load up your system with drugs. All drugs are poisonous to your cells. Different drugs have a chemical affinity for particular tissues, which is where they end up. Barbiturates are attracted to the cells in your brain stem and cortex. The cells in those parts of the brain put up a fight in an effort to get rid of the poison. With each new dose of barbiturates your cells become weaker than before. A chemical residue builds up. Instead of giving your body the rest it needs, drugs end up depleting your energy stores. In the long run they leave you more exhausted than you were to begin with.

(*Caution:* If you think you might be drug dependent, be sure to seek professional guidance before attempting to withdraw. If you're taking cortisone, barbiturates, insulin, or thyroid medication, check with your physician before either altering your dosage or attempting to withdraw from medication entirely.)

STIMULANTS KEEP YOU AWAKE WHEN YOU NEED SLEEP. Coffee, tea, amphetamines, and caffeine-laden cola drinks irritate a group of cells in your brain stem which influence the central nervous system. The irritation triggers a speedup of your thought processes and nervous responses. Your cells begin to work harder. Not getting the sleep you need, you become prey to chronic fatigue. Then you drink more coffee or take more pills to keep your responses accelerated. A vicious cycle is under way. You're drawing on precious reserves of nervous energy and courting serious exhaustion.

Clearly, these artificial means of tampering with your metabolism are bad for you. Get off the stimulants and drugs! It may be difficult for the first few days—or weeks—but remember your reason for withdrawing. *Addiction to chemicals causes you to age prematurely!* Stop the chemicals and you'll soon be giving your body the *natural* rest it needs—and adding years to your life!

Here Are Some Things You Can Do to Achieve Your Four Kinds of Rest Naturally

PHYSICAL REST

» When you're tired at the end of a day's activities, *go to bed.* Don't fight the exhaustion you feel, even if, at first, it means going to bed at eight o'clock in the evening! Your body will soon work out its own, natural schedule.

» If you're insomniac, it's especially important to give up stimulants—coffee, chocolate, tea, alcohol (for some people alcohol acts as a stimulant), and cigarettes. Foods like meat and sugary junk food are stimulating. To clear your system, fast for a day or two, and then begin eating according to the rules set forth in Your New Lifetime Eating Plan (Chapter 8). Start jogging every day, even if it's only once around the block. Go to bed at the same time every night. (Recent clinical studies of insomniacs show this to be very helpful.) Try this simple exercise to relax and slow down the system after you get into bed. Take a deep breath and hold to the count of twenty. Release, breathe normally for a minute, and repeat as often as necessary until you drop off to sleep.

MENTAL REST

» Learn a new, low-stress way of handling your problems. Instead of flying into a rage when something goes wrong, accept it as a challenge. Figure out what you can do to change the situation and solve the problem. If you can't change it, accept it and go on from there. Let it be a learning experience, something that will help you in solving future problems.

» Once a day, give yourself an affirmative pep talk. Encourage yourself. Concentrate on those things you like about yourself. Better still, write these pep talks out on paper and refer to them whenever things start to get out of hand.

SENSORY REST

» Spend a few minutes each day in a quiet place, away from noise, away from the smells of food and smoke and traffic. Have nothing to eat or drink at this time. Close your eyes and try to block out all thoughts and feelings. Imagine that your mind is nothing but a large, black screen, on which, superimposed, the numbers from 100 down to 1 appear slowly. Or choose a simple, unprovocative word and repeat it over and over again as a way of keeping other thoughts out of your consciousness. When these thoughts do sneak in, don't be upset. Just observe them, quietly, and let them drift on. *These are meditation techniques. Scientists have proved that it's possible, through meditation, to reach a state of mental and physical relaxation which is even greater than that reached during Stage IV or the deepest phase of sleep.*

» Set aside a day a week as no television or radio day. Spend that time reading poetry, walking, thinking, reading.

PHYSIOLOGICAL REST

» Set aside one day every week to give your digestive organs a rest. Fast. If you feel you can't fast, have nothing but *fresh* orange juice, fresh pineapple juice, watermelon, or freshly squeezed vegetable juice. If you're obese, arthritic, or have chronic digestive problems, skin problems, or chronic hypoglycemia, consider going to a fasting retreat for a supervised fast.

» Give up night-eating so your digestive organs can have a longer period of rest each night.

» Skip breakfast once in a while for the same reason. It extends the nightly fast.

» Cut down—or out—substances your cells can't use for your nourishment and that consequently cause more work for your excretory organs: salt, spices, vitamin pills, alcohol, drugs, coffee, and tea.
» Instead of a coffee break, have a fruit break. An apple or an orange or a bunch of sweet, ripe grapes is much easier on your digestive system than caffeine and pastry.
» Eat simple foods that leave less waste in your cells and are less work to digest: fresh ripe fruits and vegetables, seeds, whole grains.

Stop overworking your cells! By following these suggestions you'll cut down on their workload. You will also improve or expedite the natural processes of body repair and renewal. This means a more rested you, a more energetic you, a more alive you, a younger you!

It is by maintaining this proper balance between work and rest that you maintain balance and integrity within. Set aside a time for a vacation when you can leave your business or work and the physical and mental stresses connected with it. (Vacations are not luxuries; in the world we live in, they're necessities!)

Women with small children *especially* must find a way of taking a vacation from the incredibly high level of concentrated work that rearing toddlers and infants demands. You might consider a series of mini-vacations on weekends. Leave the little ones with a relative or friend and get off by yourself, with your husband. You'll return refreshed and happy. The children will benefit as well.

GETTING YOUR FULL SHARE OF NATURAL REST, REGULARLY, IS ABSOLUTELY ESSENTIAL FOR THE BORN-AGAIN BODY!

CHAPTER 19

Your Body Responds to Happiness

In certain parts of the Soviet Union, Russian peasants are living to the ripe old age of 140, 150, and sometimes even 170. (If the idea of living that long depresses you, you can be sure it's a sign that something's wrong in your life.) The Kiev Institute of Gerontology decided to conduct studies of these peasants to see what they're doing right that the rest of us might do. At the end of their research the Institute concluded that *most Americans and most Russians are living lives at least 50 years shorter than they might!*

A MAJOR FACTOR IN THE LONGEVITY OF THE UKRANIAN PEAS-ANTS WHO ARE LIVING TO 150 IS HAPPINESS.

Of course diet, too, plays a role—although scientists weren't surprised at this. The Kiev peasants eat very little fat in their diets, very little meat, don't smoke cigarettes, and don't drink alcohol—except wine! Scientists *were* surprised, however, at the vital importance of happiness and pleasure. When interviewed, the peasants said they're happy because their lives are active and productive up until the time they die. These people do not "retire" at the age of sixty or sixty-five. Rather, they begin working (often heavy work outdoors) at about the age of ten, and continue throughout life. They remain vibrant members of the community up until the very end. They eat properly, exercise strenuously, don't smoke, and . . . they feel good about themselves. They're happy!

Happiness is not only a normal condition for humans, it is an *essential* component of health and long life. You can cultivate good dietary habits, but unless you also cultivate habits of cheerfulness, joy, and contentment, your adrenal glands will have to work overtime to produce the extra amounts of adrenaline and cortisone needed to help your body cope with the stress caused by worry and unhappiness.

YOU MUST BE HAPPY TO BE HEALTHY.

William George Jordan, a former editor of the old *Saturday Evening Post*, once said: "For what man *has*, he may be dependent upon others; what he *is* rests with him alone."

Happiness is not in *having*, but in *being*.

What you *are* is what health is all about. Health means wholeness. Gladness of being can't exist unless you are a whole person, a healthy person. Wholeness—a sound mind in a sound body—is a happy state of being. It's the ultimate goal of a life fulfilled.

YOU MUST CHOOSE A HAPPY WAY OF LIFE. It is too often true, in these days we live in, that happiness doesn't just "happen." As you must choose to be thin rather than fat, and healthy rather than sick, so, too, you must choose to be happy rather than miserable. Just as thinness can't be bought or obtained through anyone's efforts but your own, neither can happiness be obtained through things or people outside yourself. You must learn to live in such a way that happiness will be yours. *This means taking charge of your thought processes and reconditioning your approach to YOU.*

FOUR COMPONENTS OF HAPPINESS ARE: GRATIFICATION, SATISFACTION, CONTENTMENT, AND PLEASURE.

1) Being able to control your own life instead of being manipulated by others is *gratifying*.

2) The attainment of self-set goals brings *satisfaction*, whether those goals have to do with worldly achievement, or achieving better health through knowledge and self-discipline, or being involved in service to others, or becoming a good artist or gardener. As you go along you'll find that once reached, your original goals will lead to new and higher ones.

3) Each step higher brings you *contentment*. Each step higher is an occasion for renewed self-pride. Warm contentment comes from the realization that you're fulfilling your plan and reaching your goal of health and happiness.

There is *pleasure* beyond compare in the satisfaction and contentment of healthful living. Some of the things you can find delightful pleasure in are:

- » Self-mastery.
- » The exquisite flavors of luscious ripe fruits and vegetables.
- » Healthy skin, clear eyes, greater vitality.
- » The soft wind in your face as you take your daily jog.
- » Waking refreshed after a restful night's sleep.
- » Your lover's touch and your healthy body's joyous response.
- » The freedom and peace of mind your new knowledge allows as you take responsibility for your own health and life.

What you must understand, however, is that not one of these pleasures all by itself will bring you happiness. Rather, together with all the other positive emotions, they form the notes and chords in the grand symphony of happiness that your life can become. Sour notes and bad chords (unhealthy living habits and negative thinking), must be eliminated in order for sweet harmony to prevail.

YOUR HAPPINESS CONTRIBUTES TO THE BETTERMENT OF *ALL* LIFE. As the components of happiness blend together into the symphony of your life, so all our lives blend together into the universal symphony. On this planet we humans suffer much discord due to our lack of awareness of the utter importance of every single note to the harmony of the whole. Each step forward you take will lead you to greater harmony and beauty, affording ultimate happiness not only for you, but lending encouragement, inspiration, and pleasure to those around you.

THE BEST WAY TO BEGIN "PROJECT HAPPINESS" IS TO GET YOUR PHYSICAL SELF IN TUNE. In 1959, one of our first guests at Pawling Manor was a pudgy, spectacled, balding grandpa from Passaic, New Jersey. His name was Sam Hilton. Sam came to lose weight but it was soon clear that his real problem was a deep-seated hopelessness about his life. He had just retired after many years in a job he liked and had come to depend on to bring meaning to his existence. Suddenly, after retiring, his total outlook on life had turned sour.

Bob and I tried our best to cheer him up. I'd take Sam with me when I went shopping. Afterward, he'd sit dejectedly in the kitchen as I made up salads and steamed vegetables and set up trays.

"Cheer up, Sam!" I'd say to him, smiling his way. "What can be so hopeless about life? You've got a terrific wife and beautiful grandchildren. You've got everything to live for!"

Sam would wrinkle his forehead, the corners of his mouth would droop into his jowls, and tears would begin to trickle and then flow from beneath his rimless spectacles. "I've got *nothing* to live for," he'd reply. "Now I'm retired, I've got nothing to do. Life is so empty, I wish I were dead."

It was a struggle to keep Sam's morale from disappearing altogether as he went through his 30 days of total fasting. The pounds began to melt away. Finally, he broke his fast. His wife came from Passaic to drive him back home. "It's going to be rough," she said, as we all helped Sam get settled into the car for his return to his retirement.

"Keep active, Sam," Bob said to him. "When you feel depressed or have nothing to do, get out and take a long walk. It's good for you!"

SMILIN' SAM—TRULY A MIRACLE! A few months later, after one of Bob's lectures in New York, a radiant, healthy, happy-looking Sam came around and handed me a card. "Smilin' Sam Hilton" were the words centered on the card. I was thrilled and amazed as Sam related his success story.

"I followed Doc's advice," he beamed. "I've kept to the regime. I've walked hundreds of miles. The more I walked the happier I got. As I began to re-cover my walking territory, I made friends along the way. Now they wait for me, and we visit and *I* encourage *them*! They call me Smilin' Sam!"

Sam got himself tuned up and tuned in by fasting, eating sensibly, and by filling up his time with physical activity. Ultimately he became an inspiration to others. The roads he walked became his road to happiness.

YOU, TOO, CAN BECOME HEALTHY AND HAPPY. Rules for getting started on your road to happiness are:

1) *Start with your physical self*, as Sam did. If you're overweight or underweight, or sluggish, suffering from chronic health problems like hypoglycemia, arthritis, constipation, skin problems, *whatever*, do begin now to eliminate the problem.

» Follow the instructions in "How to Manage a Short Fast" (Chapter 7)

» Begin, immediately thereafter, to incorporate the New Lifetime Eating Plan (Chapter 8)

» At the same time, begin the exercise plan laid out in Chapter 15.

2) Set aside a half hour each day and find a quiet, private place where you can rest your mind and body and contemplate *who you are* and *who you want to be.* Take a pen and notebook with you. Write down what your goals are for the next year. The next five years. If you haven't thought about goals:

» List the things in your life you'd like to be different.

» Make another list of ways you think you can start to change those areas of your life that keep you from being the person you'd like to be. (Try to be as realistic as possible.)

» Determine to begin work toward making these changes in your life. Determine that you will begin to be good to yourself—in a reasonable way.

» Eliminate thoughts of unpleasant things that have happened in the *past.* Dwelling on past disappointments, problems, and relationships will cause you to be depressed. Begin to live for each new day alone.

» Resolve that you will quit trying to solve all your *future* problems. Dwelling on what *might* happen, or overemphasizing your future, will create anxiety and keep you from coping successfully with today.

Each day, read over the lists you've made up and keep your objectives in the back of your mind. This may sound simplistic, but try it. You'll see that as the days and weeks go by, solutions will begin to come to you. Slowly you will generate a feeling of mastery and control over your life.

3) Actively do something every single day to improve yourself. Something that will make it easier for you to achieve your goals. If your goal is to be thin, make some change in your diet that will work toward losing weight faster—perhaps saying "no" to second helpings, or skipping lunch, or giving up desserts.

If your goal is getting a job that requires more self-confidence than you possess, sign up for a course in public relations. Buy or borrow from the library a book that can help you and begin to study that book! A good book to get you started is Napoleon Hill's *Grow Rich with Peace of Mind.*

4) *Find at least fifteen or twenty minutes a day* to get away from your daily routine and be physically active. Take a bike ride; jog around the block a few times; walk in the woods; go to the Y for a workout

or a swim. Lift weights. Jump rope. Force that sedentary, lethargic body to do, do, do. Before long, it will bring you joy!

ACCOMPLISHING THE GOALS YOU SET FORTH WILL MAKE YOU HAPPY. Fix in your mind the thought that you will persist in your search for a better, more rewarding life. As you begin following these rules and concentrating on self-improvement, you'll begin to realize that your possibilities for growth and change are infinite. The awareness of your own worth and beauty and the importance of *you* as a symbiotically necessary component of all life—the enjoyment of being a harmonious, efficiently working part of the whole rather than a sour note of discord—will bring you inner peace and happiness and the concomitant better health that goes along with that happiness.

CHAPTER 20

Born-Again Desire

Many of us, at different times in our lives, discover somewhat sadly that our sexual desire has ebbed. I say sadly, because at times like these what we experience is not anger or frustration over having our desires thwarted and our needs go unmet. At times like these we don't even *feel* our sexual needs. All we sense is the vague, discomforting notion that something's missing. Then, if we permit ourselves to dwell on the lack, the fact that our sex lives have become dull, perfunctory, or perhaps even nonexistent, will slowly rise to the level of consciousness. It is then that we feel sad, for anyone who has ever experienced deep sexual pleasure knows that the greatest natural high, the ultimate invigorator, the highest inspiration for life is love for another human. The merging of spirits as well as bodies brings exquisite pleasure quite beyond description. It is an electrical experience that gives special meaning to life and makes it totally worthwhile.

Once the passion of adolescence subsides and we take up our adult lives, it's all too easy to become caught up in work and worry and turn off to our physical selves. Wanting to be "responsible" we dive into our work, our childrearing, and all the adult chores of life with a vengeance. Perhaps you're in this sexual limbo right now. Perhaps you've been there for some time. It makes no difference. It's still possible to turn things around. You can enjoy the electrical phenomenon that I call total sex on into a physical age that defies conventional acceptance. It may not and need not be a daily part of your life, but when it happens you'll be glad you're healthy and alive. Total sex is the ultimate payoff of good health.

IF YOU'RE AT A POINT IN YOUR LIFE WHERE SEX NO LONGER GIVES YOU THE PLEASURE IT ONCE DID THERE ARE SOME DEFINITE THINGS YOU CAN DO TO CHANGE THE SITUATION. I decided to talk about sex in this book because it's a book about total health and fitness and I believe that a good, strong sexual drive is the right and privilege of every healthy individual. Sexual pleasure is what we were designed for. It's part of nature's plan, just as health is. And just as you can make changes in your life to turn yourself around and become a healthy, vigorous new person, so too can you make changes that will improve your sex life. In fact, much of what you do for your body and for your health will automatically improve your sex life, as we will see. But there are mental attitudes that can stand in the way.

LET'S TALK FOR A MOMENT ABOUT PLEASURE. Everything we do in our daily lives really should be geared to our own pleasure. This is an idea that deep down we still resist, even though we may give lip service to it. Fun is fun and everybody needs a little on Saturday night, but pleasure every day? Pleasure that's *planned* for, *thought* about, even *counted* on? No, that's too much. It goes against our Puritan ideals. And yet, when you think about it, what *else* is life all about? Pain, sacrifice, struggle—obviously these come into the lives of everyone, man, woman, or child. We expect life to be difficult and we try to develop our characters in order to deal with it, but we shouldn't devote ourselves to difficulty. Pleasure should be the goal. That's right. Pleasure is what keeps us young, happy and energetic. Pleasure is what makes us *creative*. Even our most abstract scientists, philosophers, and mathematicians experience the keenest pleasure in what they do. Einstein may have been a genius but he never would have been the inventor he was without his innate love of life.

Think, for a moment, of the happiest people you know. It could be an insurance salesman who bounds out of bed every morning for a two-mile run before going to work. It could be the woman in your office who has energy for everything and is always so alive looking and full of exuberance. It's not a question of what these people do for a living, or how old they are, or how much education they've had. If they're happy they all beam out the same message to the world: *I feel good. I enjoy life. I love what I am doing.*

People who feel this way almost invariably have positive attitudes toward their bodies and actively pursue good health. These same people almost invariably enjoy good sex lives. It's co-axiomatic. You can't have good sex without caring for and respecting your total self, and you can't care for and respect your total self without having good, satisfying sex. (Some, of course, choose *not* to express themselves sexually because of a particular cause or ideal they're living for, but these people are exceptions; also, their capacity for deep sexual pleasure is always there, as long as they're otherwise healthy.)

What I'm talking about, again, is *wholeness.* We are thinking, feeling beings and we are physical, sexual beings. To deny ourselves sexual pleasure is the same as to deny our intellects the chance to function at peak capacity. To deny ourselves sexual pleasure is the same as to deny ourselves the right to feel our feelings.

ONLY WHEN WE GRASP THE *RIGHTNESS* OF SEXUAL PLEASURE WILL WE BE FREE TO PURSUE IT. And we *should* pursue it, as actively as we pursue good health. Ask yourself these questions:

Do I have the right to a good sex life?

Am I proud of my sexual feelings?

Are my sexual experiences as good, as frequent and as intense as I'd like them to be?

If your answer to any one of these questions isn't an exhilarated "Yes!," then you have some changes to make. The first change is to assert the goodness of your own sexuality to yourself. Say, "I have the right to good, strong sexual pleasure and I want it." That's right, say it out loud in a room by yourself. If you feel insecure about it, it's a clear indication that you're squeamish about your sexual needs. At the risk of feeling silly, do as I say and repeat the phrase, only louder this time: *"I have the right to good, strong sexual pleasure and I want it."*

That may feel a little scary. When we begin to assert our needs they become more conscious, and with that comes the realization that we have to *do* something about them. ("Who me?" a little voice inside you counters.) All right, now you're going to blast it out with the same vehemence that you'd assert your right to be yourself. I HAVE THE RIGHT TO GOOD, STRONG SEXUAL PLEASURE AND I WANT IT! If you didn't manage to yell that out with the entire fullness of your being, do it again. You should find yourself experiencing a little quiver of returning life. Yell it out until you do, and don't be afraid of that feeling. Be joyful! It means those delicious sexual feelings will come surging to you in abundance.

Accepting our sexuality is absolutely necessary if we're going to open the floodgates of sexual pleasure but there are also specific, physical measures to take that will help to bring you back in tune with your sexual self. They are the same things that will bring you to a condition of general fitness and health.

1) *Raise your level of natural energy* with a diet high in natural carbohydrates and low in protein—especially fatigue-inducing animal protein. You can't have good sex when you're tired, draggy or sick. You need a high level of ready energy, the sort you get from natural sugars.

2) *Put your body into shape with exercise.* Unrelieved mental activity or a job that's solely sedentary can easily put you out of touch with your body. Exercise will begin to make you *feel* yourself again: your legs, your arms, your neck, the small of your back. Do your exercises in front of a full-length mirror and revel in your body and the sensations it generates as you move and bend. If these sensations should become sexual, let them. Use exercise to allow yourself the opportunity of giving full vent to your natural feelings.

3) *Get more rest.* Give yourself the chance for calm, luxuriant rest and relaxation. If you're feeling tense and overworked, try retiring earlier in the evening. Make your baths longer, warmer, and more thoughtless. Let yourself become *de-stimulated,* mentally, and your body will begin to take over. Enjoy the way your limbs glisten in the water. Rest your head on the back of the tub and get into the sensation of floating.

THE FOOD-SEX CONNECTION. There's a strong relationship between food and sex. As infants our earliest form of gratification was the nourishment we received at mother's breast. The food-sex connection was forged almost as soon as we were born, and it continues to influence us as long as we're alive. Because of it, most people use food as a sex substitute at various times in their lives. If you're feeling insecure about yourself, it's safe to go to the refrigerator. There, without having to feel emotionally vulnerable to another person, you can just help your self and then shut the door.

One sure way to douse the flame of your sexual ardor is to overeat. People with a tendency to do this often do it unconsciously. It keeps them from feeling anxious about sex and about their natural drive for sexual pleasure. It keeps them from feeling anxious about needing something from someone else. At the Manor we've noticed that many of the overweight women who come to fast find themselves experiencing an almost alarming desire for sex. Their food has been taken away from them! Their natural sex drive has a chance to come to the surface and flourish again.

Men, too, have reported more and stronger erections, although men tend to experience their renewed sexual drive after the fast is over, rather than during it.

FASTING AND THE SEX RESPONSE. The complete physiological vacation your body gets during a fast affects every part of it, including the sex organs. Fasting invigorates and refreshes all the cells in the body, paving the way for a renewed response to life— and that includes a renewed sexual response. One woman who loved her husband very much but had been sexually turned off for over a year came to Pawling Health Manor to fast and lose weight. An unexpected result of her fast was the renewal of her desire for her husband. At the end of only a week without food she felt like a different person. I found the letter she wrote to me when she got home very touching.

Dear Joy,

There's never been any doubt that I love my husband, Bill, but for a long time now I've had hardly any interest in sex. I know it's been painful for Bill because he could sense my disinterest and it made him feel inadequate. I would make love whenever he wanted, but I never wanted. He knew it, I knew it, and it was making us both very unhappy.

When I came to Pawling to fast it was to lose weight. Lose weight I did (twelve pounds in a week) but I never expected what happened afterward. When I got home I stayed off the junk food and ate mainly the fruits and vegetables, as you recommended. Then, surprise of surprises, after a couple of weeks I found myself getting . . . well, I hate to say it, but horny! *At first I was almost embarrassed. (I hadn't yet lost all the weight I needed to lose. Also, it had been so* long. *Would my husband still want me? Would he reject me?) But Bill, bless him, was overjoyed. Our relationship is on a new level now. I feel better in every way, but what makes me happiest is to feel like a complete, sexual person again.*

Love,
Renata S.

The P.S. to this story is that six months later Renata came back for another fast, and now she looks as vibrant and sexy as she feels.

What happened to Renata happens to many women who decide to change the way they eat. The fast undoubtedly helps, because it gets the body into a cleaner state. After fasting you're particularly responsive to the benefits of eating a diet high in natural carbohydrates, especially fresh fruits and vegetables. Your general health improves radically, your energy level soars, and very often your sexual drive will come back with all the force and beauty it had when you first became aware of sexual feelings as a teenager. *That's the way natural sex feels:* strong, thrilling, and beautiful. It's very different from the artificially induced sensations brought on by stimulating foods, alcohol, drugs. The reason pornography is so big in our society today is because people have lost much of their normal sex feeling, or desire, and they have to prod themselves visually into the same kinds of feelings that would surface spontaneously if they were living natural lives.

A DIET HIGH IN ARTIFICIAL FOODS CAUSES THE METABOLISM TO SPEED UP IN ORDER TO GET RID OF THEM AND ULTIMATELY DEPRESSES SEXUAL FUNCTIONING. Healthy sex is like healthy food. You may think that processed, sugary, or highly spiced and salted foods taste good while you're eating them, but you won't know until you've fasted and broken your addiction to these foods that *natural* foods can taste so superfantastic it's unimaginable. Good sex, like good food, is a matter of *quality,* not quantity.

Premature sexual dysfunction, like premature aging, is brought on by a poor diet. It's possible to be quite active sexually *not* because you're in touch with genuine, healthy sexual instincts, but because your life is filled with artificial stimulation. If you always drink before sex, for example, your sex drive is being artificially jogged. You may have the momentary pleasure of the orgasm but over the long run you're putting your body under terrific stress. Everything you do that causes your cells to age sooner than they should wears down your whole system. Your natural sex drive and sex function will be affected prematurely by a hard-driving, unnatural lifestyle, just as the rest of your body will be.

FASTING AND A DIET OF NATURAL FOODS HAVE OFTEN BEEN HELPFUL IN FERTILITY PROBLEMS. Herbert Shelton says that fasting has helped many women to conceive after years of sterility.

Over the years, women have gone to his fasting institute in Texas with a history of menstrual irregularities, profuse flow, severe cramps that send them to bed each month, large clots, soreness of the breasts, and similar symptoms that indicate endocrine (ductless gland) imbalance or inflammation of the ovaries or womb. Others gave a history of more or less chronic vaginal discharge whose acid content was sufficient to destroy the sperm. "These are the types of cases that are most readily corrected and that are restored to health by a period of physical, mental and physiological rest," Shelton wrote in *Fasting Can Save Your Life*. "Few cases of female infertility are absolute; most of them are the outgrowth of conditions of disease and are remediable. Great numbers of women have found the ability to conceive restored by a return to good health, and a large part of these women have found the fast of inestimable value in the clearing up of conditions that prevented conception."

There's a story of a husband and wife that I'd like to share with you because it sums up a lot of what we've talked about in this chapter. Martin Gray lived an extraordinary life, having been in nine concentration camps before he was fourteen years of age. His entire family was wiped out in the Holocaust and it was many years of scratching for survival before he met his wife, Dina. Doctors said Dina's only chance of having children was surgery. Martin didn't want that. Then they met a couple with a history of fertility problems. The wife had finally conceived after fasting and changing her diet. In a beautiful book he wrote about his life, called *For Those I Loved*, Martin Gray describes what happened after coming to Pawling Health Manor to fast.

I was a regular customer at Manny Wolf's Chop House. I used to bolt down hamburgers at P.J. Clark's, the famous restaurant on Third Avenue (in New York). I'd lived on vodka, even drunk raw alcohol in the perfume factory. I was a red-meat eater. All that changed in days. Dina dragged me to meetings and, in the mornings, read out loud from books on health foods and vegetarianism.

"Nature, Martin. Let's have a natural life."

We gave up smoking. We were happy, strong, united; we were building our own life, we were discovering it together. We'd sacrificed what had been meager, lonely pleasures to commune together, in certainty. We gave up meat and salt and lived on nuts, grapefruit, and bananas.

"I feel good, Martin. I feel light."

We were bringing each other back to life. Dina went on a two-week fast in Dr. Gross's clinic. I stayed with her, served her tumblers of grapefruit juice, watched her sleeping, saw her growing younger. A month later, she was pregnant.

"You see!"

She was up against me, so soft, her skin so smooth. I kissed her; stroked her belly: life was there, her life and mine. I wanted to change myself, too. I began a long fast. Lying down, eyes half closed, I felt transformed. Dr. Gross told me to sleep but how could I when my brain had never been so active. I sought the meaning of our life there, in the sunshine, the children around us who would grow to be real men. I fasted for thirty-eight days. Colleagues phoned Gross, phoned Dina: "Stop him! He'll die!"

I was reborn. I shook off the dust of the ghetto, the yellow sand and sweat of Treblinka, the mud of the Polish forests and the dried blood that had stuck to my hands. I lost thirty-eight pounds. I never felt so young: my bones, my muscles, that had been beaten and wrenched so many times had gained another suppleness.

"You're very thin," said Dina, "all clean and new."

. . .

I wasn't permitted to see Nicole being born. I waited with a few others in the large hall of Doctors' Hospital in Manhattan. Hedy and Felix Gluckselig, Viennese antique dealers whom Dina had introduced to me, were there and tried joking with me.

"You're like all husbands," said Hedy.

She held my hands, tried to calm me, but she realized that this birth meant even more to me than to most fathers. Through it my people would live again.

A nurse came at last, with a big smile.

"It's a girl."

Thank you, Dina. From them, from me.

YOUR
30-DAY
BORN-AGAIN
BODY PROGRAM

CHAPTER 21

30 Days
to a New You

The beauty of this 30-day plan lies in its utter simplicity. As you get into it you'll find new awareness and enjoyment in the simple pleasures of daily living. You will experience new, natural "highs" that will astound you. The fantastic pleasure you'll get from your first sip of orange juice after your first fast is only the beginning.

You don't have to change all your eating habits immediately. It takes time to reach your ideals. The Born-Again Body Program is meant to get you going. It's an intense "rejuvenation special" to show you that it *can* be done and that the results will be fantastic.

It's important not to give up if you slip from time to time. We *all* slip. If you should go off on a food binge now and again, don't let it get the better of you. Put your mind back in charge, reprogram your computer, and become your own boss once again. Start each day afresh, forgetting yesterday's hassles. Don't worry about the temptations you may have tomorrow. Live each day for itself. Day by day you'll come closer to your true self, that terrific person who was there all the time but couldn't get out!

Your 30-day program begins with a three-day fast, if you are employed outside, or a four-day fast if you're at home. This mini-fast is necessary to clean out some of the debris or toxic material that's accumulated in your system, and to improve your body chemistry. It will get you off to a flying start. You will learn, gently and easily, how to get on and come off a fast. You'll also learn how marvelous fasting makes you look and feel.

During the rest of the month you'll be learning how to eat according to your New Lifetime Eating Plan. By following this program you will *automatically* learn what foods you should be eating and in what quantities, and how you should combine them.

Depending upon your individual metabolism, and your weight when starting the program, you can lose from ten to twenty pounds in about a month's time—if weight loss is among the things you're after. If you *don't* want to lose weight but are simply looking for new energy and rejuvenation, you can follow the modified, non-weight-loss guidelines.

One last reminder before you begin. Expect to feel a "low" when you first give up the coffee, sugar, meat, and other stimulating foods you're accustomed to. Once your system adjusts, you'll be quite "high" on your own sense of well-being. Ordinarily, this change-over from artificially induced to natural high takes place in a matter of days. Just don't let that initial "low" deter you. Consider it a good sign—an indication that your body is getting off the toxins that have been aging you before your time. The "low" means you are in the vital detoxification stage of your Born-Again Program. Once this initial but unavoidable "low" is over, it's all uphill. Your body will begin to stream with new tingling sensations of energy and vitality. As you master each day of your 30-day program, you'll begin feeling cleaner, more optimistic, *higher*—until one day, toward the end of the month, you will actually wake up feeling as though you've been born again.

MANY PEOPLE FIND IT VERY HELPFUL TO KEEP A JOURNAL WHILE THEY ARE ON THIS PROGRAM. They note weight loss, physical changes and reactions, thoughts about the present and future as they feel themselves changing, and any inspirational or practical ideas that occur along the way. I'll tell you more about this as we go through the program together.

DAY ONE

Headset

Today and every day for the duration of the program, you're going to have an evaluating talk with yourself before you get out of bed. This daily dialogue will help you to be more aware of how you're thinking and feeling. By raising your awareness of yourself, the morning dialogue will help you to put your mind in charge of your actions for the day.

1) Today, create a mental picture of yourself the way you'd like to be. Think of how you'd like to look, how you'd like to feel, physically, and how you'd like to feel about yourself. Concentrate on that image for thirty seconds.

2) Imagine that inside your brain there's a panel of control buttons. One button is labeled "Kind of Food," one "Amount of Food," one "Fasting," one "Exercise." You can create as many "buttons" as you think will be helpful to you in controlling your daily actions.

3) Tell yourself that instead of allowing these buttons to be operated by remote controls originating in the brains of food advertising executives and other vested interests, you are going to operate your own buttons—when and how you choose.

4) Today, push the "Fasting" button. Say to yourself, "I'm going to begin a fast today that will cleanse my body of toxins and help it to respond to the new, healthy foods I'm going to begin eating. I will become the attractive, healthy person I want to be."

Exercise

Today you'll do some mild stretching and bending exercises. Stand on your toes, arms straight up overhead, fingers touching. Pretend you're trying to touch the ceiling.

With your feet about twelve inches apart, hands clasped together (arms still overhead), upper torso straight, bend to the left and s-t-r-e-t-c-h as though trying to touch the floor with the sides of your head. Gently staighten up to your starting position. Repeat 4 times.

Now bend to the right and repeat 4 times.

Lean forward. Keeping your knees straight, try to touch the floor with your fingertips. Bounce forward 10 times. Feel the pull in the back of your legs.

Run in place for 2 minutes, or until you begin to breathe deeply and rhythmically.

Natural grooming tip

Good grooming is essential to help you look and feel as good about yourself as possible. While the most important aspect of changing your health is changing from the *inside*, it's good to care properly for the outside of you, too. On some days I'll be passing along tips for natural grooming that I've found helpful through the years. I'll be encouraging you to use simple, non-chemical products in place of commercial ones.

Eating plan

Breakfast, lunch, and dinner today is water. You can have it hot, cold, or tepid. If you feel rumbling going on in your stomach when it doesn't get its accustomed food, don't be disturbed. Once your digestive system adjusts to fasting the rumbling will stop. Let the information in Chapter 7 be a guide during this week.

Night thought

Feel *proud* for having stuck to your plan for the day. YOU ARE WONDERFUL! Meditate on these words:

> If one advances confidently in the direction of his dreams and endeavors to live the life which he has imagined, he will meet with success unexpected in common hours.
>
> —HENRY DAVID THOREAU

DAY TWO

Headset

Before you get up have your morning talk with yourself. Think for a moment about yesterday's successful fasting. You feel lighter and thinner already. Be proud of your accomplishment!

» In your journal, write down your current chest, waist, and hip measurements.
» Study your posture. Are you happy with it? Write down your evaluation.

You will check back with your notes seven days from now, and once a week for the remainder of the month. Plan to use this notebook as a tool for improving yourself.

Exercise

Today, skip calisthenics to conserve energy for the housecleaning activity the fast is producing inside of you. If you feel slightly headachy or nauseous, don't worry. It won't last long and it's par for the course. It means you're coming off your food and coffee high and your body is reacting. You may throw up some low-grade bile.

Natural grooming tip

Don't shower if you feel tired. Take a sponge bath with tepid water. Some people find hot water too enervating when they fast.

Eating plan

Morning: Water. Don't drink any more than your natural thirst demands.
Lunch: Water. Sip it slowly.
Dinner: Get out a pretty teacup and saucer. Pour yourself a cup of hot water and sip it slowly, a teaspoonful at a time, until it cools sufficiently to drink from the cup. Notice how your sense of smell has improved. You are acutely aware of smells not only of food, but of the fresh air and growing things.

Night Thought

Take a warm, slow, luxurious bath and go to bed. Feel *proud* of yourself for having succeeded with this, your second day of fasting. You are really beginning to take charge of your life.

> Living structure is obedient to the mind.
> —HERBERT SHELTON

DAY THREE

Headset

Today, on the third day of your fast, your morning date with the scale is encouraging. You've lost from three to five pounds. Make a note of this in your Born-Again notebook.

By this time you may be feeling uncomfortable, a little restless, preoccupied with thoughts of food, headachy. Write down any such symptoms you might have, as you're trying to reconstruct a record of this whole rejuvenating adventure. Tell yourself, "These are good signs—it means I'm breaking the food habit. Tomorrow I'll feel much better!"

Exercise

No exercise today. If you find yourself feeling a bit restless, don't worry, it's a normal reaction. By now your brain's glucose supply is lower than normal. For this reason take care not to get up too suddenly—you may get dizzy. Move slowly.

Remember also that the less active you are, the more energy reserve there is for your internal cleaning out process and the better your final results will be.

Natural grooming tip

Today have your hairdresser or a friend do your hair. It's best not to shampoo your own, as the effort of arms over head can be tiring when you're fasting.

Eating plan

Water again, and only if you're thirsty and feel the need for it. When you're not eating, you need less water than usual.

If water begins to taste unpleasant it's because your sense of taste is heightened during a fast. Impurities in most conventional water supplies will become more noticeable. Distilled water (you can get it at a drug store) should help solve the problem.

Night thought

If you feel more energetic this evening (this sometimes happens as a fast progresses), go to a movie or take a drive in the car. But make an early evening of it. As you relax into sleep tonight, you should feel very pleased with yourself. *You are in control.*

> Each of us is the leader of his or her own liberation.
> —CHARLES REICH

DAY FOUR

Headset

To get your head set for today, take out your notebook and list the ways in which you're beginning to *look better* and *feel better*. You're a pound or two lighter, even, than yesterday. Your eyes are brighter. Your skin is clearer. You're one step closer to the real, the new, you.

Exercise

Continue conserving your energy today. Soon enough you'll be into a vigorous, new exercise regime.

Food Plan

If you're not going to work, stick to pure water this one last day.

If you *are* employed outside, today you'll begin to eat again. Here's your re-feeding plan:

Breakfast:
Watermelon wedge (2″ × 6″)
Lunch:
Two juicy ripe oranges
Dinner:
Large bunch of seedless white grapes
or
Two pieces of citrus fruit
or
10 ounces of celemato
Celemato: Cut two or three ripe tomatoes in wedges and put into blender. Turn on high and push pieces down in with a large stalk of green celery. Pour into a tall glass. Sip slowly or eat with a soupspoon.

If you *must* eat lunch in a restaurant today, have your citrus fruit in the morning and order melon at the restaurant. Watermelon is preferable, but if it's not available, order any fresh, ripe melon—cantaloupe, honeydew, or Spanish. If the restaurant has no melon, ask for a fresh tomato salad without dressing.

Night thought

Be proud that you're helping yourself rejuvenate through fasting. Before going to sleep tonight, contemplate this mandala. It will help you to focus on the wholeness and integrity of the new life you're beginning.

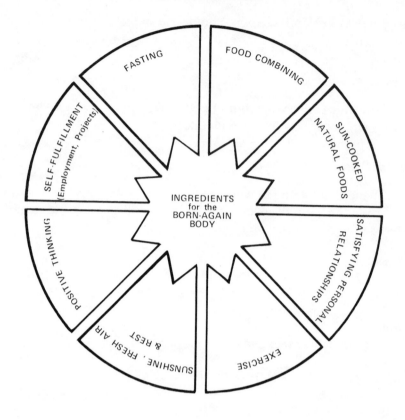

One sees things in fragments and thinks in fragments.
We must inquire into what it means to see totally.

—J. KRISHNAMURTI

DAY FIVE

Headset

Write in your notebook: I am going to eat *only* what's prescribed, today and every other day of my Born-Again Program.

Look yourself over in the mirror. Write down areas of your
body you think will need special work when you begin your exercise regimen tomorrow.

Exercise

As a reward for your self-discipline during the fast, arrange that
a husband, lover, or friend give you a massage today. Use the following instructions as a guide:

1) Pull your hair back into a scarf or small towel for protection.

2) Have ready 4 ounces of safflower, almond, or other cold pressed oil.

3) Lie down on a flat surface, such as a bed, on which a large towel or folded sheet has been spread.

FOR THE MASSEUR OR MASSEUSE:

» Start with the face. Smooth on the oil gently and wipe off excess with tissues. Starting in the center of the eyebrows, massage very gently, kneading forehead skin away from the tension area.

» With fingertips, stroke beneath the chin and up toward ears. Repeat 6 times.

» Beginning along the jawline, make little circles with fingertips, moving up to the cheekbones. Repeat 6 times.

» Apply a thin layer of oil to the entire body, gently kneading with the palms and paying particular attention to the stomach and thigh area. Do each arm and hand. Massage each finger with a gentle twisting motion from base to tip.

» Massage the soles of the feet as firmly as possible. Stroke their tops. Massage each toe in the same fashion as the fingers.

» Turn the individual over. Massage the neck, the back, and each leg, ending with toes.

Natural grooming tip

Start thinking about revising your wardrobe. You'll soon be taking in skirts and slacks that are baggy. Discard items that clutter your closet, and put in your notebook a list of garments that need alteration.

Food plan

If you don't go to work and are breaking your fast today:

Breakfast:
One grapefruit
or
Two oranges
or
A medium-sized piece of watermelon
Lunch:
Half a ripe honeydew melon
or

Two ripe tomatoes
> *or*

8 ounces fresh orange juice
Dinner:
An orange and a grapefruit
> *or*

A large cup of vegetable broth
> *or*

A generous portion of melon

If you go to business:

Breakfast:
8 ounces fresh orange juice
2 ounces sunflower seeds
Lunch:
2 tomatoes, 1 stalk celery, 4 oz. cottage cheese. Pack the cottage cheese in a covered container, the vegetables in plastic bags, and take with you in your bag. If you don't want to pack a lunch, order a large tossed salad and a side order of cottage cheese at the restaurant.
Dinner:
Large Finger Salad
1 cup steamed kale
1 cup steamed butternut squash
6 asparagus spears

Night thought

Tonight you should feel proud of yourself not only for having adhered to your re-feeding plan for the day, but for having the determination to continue. You are truly getting yourself together.

> Getting it all together is what joy needs to operate. For whatever the cause, joy is preceded by that swift organization of parts into a whole, where suddenly what we thought was a dream translates itself into a reality . . .
>
> —PHYLLIS THOREAX
> —New York *Times*

DAY SIX

Headset

As you get into shape, you must begin to set new lifetime goals for yourself. Get out your journal and *write down* your dreams of the things you'd like to accomplish. Beginning today, do something every day that will help you realize one of your goals.

Exercise

Since you've just broken your fast, rest fifteen or twenty minutes after breakfast before you begin exercising. Then turn to p. 147 and do Exercises 1 through 10, *only*, of Yvonne's Head-to-Toe Shape-Up Program.

Food Plan

Breakfast:
   2 oranges, 12 raw cashews
Lunch:*
   A large bunch of seedless white grapes
   3 large nectarines, 3 dried figs
Dinner:
   Large Finger Salad, 1 cup fresh green peas. 1 medium-sized baked potato (including the jacket), 1 small pat of butter
Snack:
   1 large ripe banana.

Night thought

Before you go to sleep tonight, breathe deeply and think about the good day you've had. It's gratifying to know that this marvelous sense of well-being you're experiencing is happening because you've done something in your life to make it happen!

> If your life is better, it is because you have done something constructive to make it better.
> —DR. WAYNE W. DYER

---

*If you're a business person, take your grapes and nectarines with you. Or, if you eat out, order a fresh fruit salad with *no* dressing.

DAY SEVEN

Headset

Use your quiet time this morning to reinforce your goals and your new self-image. Check your weight on the scale. Read through your journal, beginning with Day One and up until the present, to see how you've progressed. You are now one week into your 30-day program! Write a paragraph in your notebook describing how you feel about yourself today.

Exercise

Before you get out of bed, go through Yvonne's antistress exercise (p. 158). Then do the stretching and loosening up techniques described on Day One. Once you feel pleasantly limber, proceed with Yvonne's Head-to-Toe Shape-Up, doing all the exercises from 1 through 20.

Natural grooming tip

For a simple, natural rinse after your shampoo this morning, use the juice of half a lemon squeezed into a quart of warm water.

Food Plan

Choose your breakfast, lunch, and dinner for today from any of the meals listed in the Month of Menus that begins on page 119.

Night thought

You have just concluded the first week of your Born-Again Body Program. There's much to feel good about. What control you are gaining, what mastery over each of life's precious days! You are learning to live truly and consciously.

> There is no need to be afraid of death. . . . Rather,
> our concern must be to *live* while we're alive!
> —ELISABETH KÜBLER-ROSS

DAY EIGHT

Headset

Here is a way to increase your ability to concentrate which makes use of the clock on your night table. Before getting out of bed this morning, sit upright with a clock at eye level. Fix your gaze on the tip of the second hand. Follow it as it sweeps around the clock face. Each time you exhale, feel your gaze focusing more and more intensely on the tip of the second hand. See if you can do this for 2 minutes without having any extraneous thoughts. If you have one, stop, rest your eyes a moment, and try again. This meditation technique will refresh you, and will help you develop the powers of the mind you need for taking fresh control of your life.

Exercise

Today, go through Yvonne's entire Head-to-Toe Shape-Up Plan, from Exercises 1 to 20.

Go outside for a short, slow run around the block or down the street you live on. If you aren't able to get out of doors, run in place in your bedroom, or jump rope for 2 minutes. (Jumping rope is more strenuous than you think.)

Natural grooming tip

When taking your bath today, put some herbs in a piece of cheesecloth and tie it on the bathtub faucet so the water can flow through it. The herbal steam created will both relax you and loosen clogged facial pores.

Food Plan

Breakfast:
    1 medium-sized apple
    8 top quality dates
Lunch:
    Sunburst Salad (See recipe in Chapter 12)
    1 cup steamed green beans
    ½ cup ricotta cheese
Dinner:
    Mixed green salad

1 cup green peas

1 cup Kentucky-Style Corn (See recipe in Chapter 13)

(Remember that if you *don't* have a weight problem you can have seconds.)

Night thought

Feel proud that today you stuck to simple foods and that you're learning to develop new body awareness. Go to sleep with a pleasant anticipation of tomorrow and its challenges.

> It's an exciting and rewarding experience to break down the bars of your custom-and-tradition cage and enjoy the freedom of the wide open spaces of the world of reason.
>
> —ROBERT J. RINGER

DAY NINE

Headset

Today makes the ninth day since you've begun instituting changes in your life. Take a mental inventory. Get out your journal and check off the goals you've reached so far.

Exercise

After going through Yvonne's Head-to-Toe Shape-Up Program, stand nude in front of your full-length mirror and give yourself a good sizing up. Now that you've lost pounds and are toning up, reexamine yourself for trouble spots. Today, pick one trouble area (thighs, upper arms, or whatever) and *do extra repetitions* of the special exercise Yvonne gives for this problem spot.

Food Plan

Today is Saturday. Treat yourself to dinner in a restaurant. It's fun and easy to dine out and still stick with your new eating plan. The most important thing is to stoke up your determination before you leave the house. Then, at the restaurant, take up the challenge of choosing a few healthful but delicious foods from the menu. Try a meal of salad, eggplant, and vegetables; or salad, baked potato, and vegetables.

Night thought

> When our senses expand we perceive the One.
> When our senses contract we perceive the Division.
> —WILLIAM BLAKE

DAY TEN

Headset

Get set for today by writing in your journal: Today I am going to do three things that will help me to grow in the new life I'm seeking!

1) Buy a copy of *Health for the Millions*, by Herbert Shelton.

2) Give up television this evening and go for a walk instead.

3) Skip lunch and stick strictly to the breakfast and dinner given in today's menu.

Do all three.

Exercise

Stand in front of the mirror, inhale deeply through your nostrils, and lean forward, hands on the front of your thighs. Blow out all your breath through your mouth and lock your breathing into HOLD position. If you take in air it will break the vacuum you've created inside you. Suck in your stomach (still without breathing), let it in and out a couple of times, and NOW, still without breathing, concentrate on isolating the two muscles that run from under your ribs down into your groin. Tense and release! Take in air, exhale, and repeat. If you keep working on this, a little each day, you'll find it will help firm up your stomach beautifully and will make you feel relaxed and conscious of the inside of your body.

Do all 20 exercises in the Head-to-Toe Program.

Natural grooming tip

Rub a blend of cold-pressed almond and sesame oils into your hands gently (you can pick these up in a health food store). Let it soak in for five minutes before wiping the excess off with a tissue.

After the oil treatment, file and shape your nails and protect them with clear polish.

Food Plan

Choose today's menus from any of the ones listed in Chapter 14.

Have a glass of Green Goddess in midmorning (recipe on page 112) or after work.

Night thought

Famous models and actresses—the beautiful people—have learned to use the power inherent within themselves. The challenge and action of its application in their lives makes them exciting people.

> There is no beauty without discipline; you must have rules. An undisciplined woman shows her disinterest in life . . . and when there is nothing behind her facade of beauty, she is boring.
>
> —BIANCA JAGGER
> —*Vogue*

DAY ELEVEN

Headset

As you get set for today, think of this 30-day plan as a training course for the future. Before you get up and become involved with your day, write the following principles down in your notebook.

1) There are certain immutable laws that govern life and health. When these laws are broken, disharmony and disease result.

2) High protein consumption forces your body to waste energy and age prematurely.

3) It's as easy to become enslaved to good habits as bad ones.

Internalizing the principles of good health will give you confidence to resist gimmicks and fads and to take charge of your body and your life.

Exercise

Today, when going through the exercises, study the photographs. Make an effort to duplicate Yvonne's movements, her balance, her poise.

Natural grooming tip

Give yourself a good all-over massage today with a loufa. Massage your body first with a light oil—baby, sesame, or almond—and then loufa yourself, giving extra massaging to the abdomen, back "wings," upper and lower underarms and thighs.

Food Plan

Today you will put the Mono-meal plan into practice. (See page 68.)

Breakfast:
1 whole Spanish (or honeydew) melon
Lunch:
Several bunches of seedless white grapes, or any type you prefer
Dinner:
All the salad you want (Choose one from Chapter 12.)

If you have a special digestive problem and can't handle the all-raw diet yet, here's a plan for you:

Breakfast:
Two or three ripe bananas
Lunch:
Two large whole baked apples
Dinner:
A large bowl of blended green salad

Night thought

Feel pleased with the progress and flexibility you've shown. Drift happily into sleep.

> The rigid never grow.
> —ROBERT J. RINGER

DAY TWELVE

Headset

During this morning's think time, concentrate on the role *struggle* is playing in the new plan for your life. Struggles are a part of your decision-making, they're those silent little battles you go through with yourself when you make choices. When you make good choices, these struggles make you strong and masterful. You've chosen well and won the struggle when you say "no" to junk food and when you say "yes" to exercise in the open air; when you say "no" to cigarettes and "yes" to a needed trip to the country or seashore. Every right choice is a seed planted for your vibrant future. Each one will ripen into a new and wonderful happening.

Exercise

Any activity that causes you to breathe deeply over a sustained period of time (a minimum of 5 minutes) will keep your heart strong and healthy if you do it regularly. Get out of doors for your aerobic exercise today. Run a mile or jump rope for 5 minutes. And of course, start your day with the Head-to-Toe Exercises that you're now able to do without turning back to Chapter 15.

Natural grooming tip

Here is an internal cleansing technique that I've practiced for thirty years. It has saved me lots of dollars and has spared my sensitive vaginal membranes from the harsh chemicals and irritants of commercial douches. I call it my "internal bath." While sitting in a tub of warm-to-hot water, use your forefinger to open the entrance of your vagina. Take a deep breath through your nostrils and blow the air out through your mouth, emptying out completely. *Without taking a breath*, suck in. You'll find that this allows water to fill your vagina. By controlling your vaginal muscles, you can swish the warm, soothing, cleansing water in and out. You mustn't breathe while doing it; if there's air inside you, it won't work. (You've already learned the beginning techniques of working your internal organs without breathing on page 207.) This is not only a natural way to cleanse this important area of your body, but a wonderful exercise that will improve your control over vaginal muscles.

Food Plan

Choose your meals today from the menus in Chapter 14.

Night thought

Before you go to sleep, reflect on the reasons why you've decided to change to a more positive lifestyle. You want to feel good. You want a more productive life. Maybe you want to set a better example for those who may depend on you for guidance. Never forget, though, that the primary reason you're changing is to make your life more enjoyable.

> Let your pleasures be real,
> not merely conventional.
> —C. G. L. DUCANN

DAY THIRTEEN

Headset

Get in the habit of clarifying for yourself what you're trying to accomplish. It will help to keep your determination bolstered. Write in your Born-Again journal:

> I will discontinue those habits that subtract from the quality of my life. I will never lose my sense of the significance and urgency of my life. I *will* live for health, beauty, joy, and productive pleasure. I won't allow myself to become less than I can be. Life is irreplaceable. *My* life is irreplaceable.

Exercise

Today, add to *all* the repetitions of your Head-to-Toe Exercises. Each day you should be giving slightly more time to your workout.

Natural grooming tip

Mix equal parts of cornmeal and oatmeal with just enough water to make a paste. Use this as a facial scrub. The grittiness will open your pores and improve circulation. Keep the mixture in a small covered jar and use once a week.

Food Plan

Here's your menu for today:

Breakfast:
3 ripe peaches, ½ cup ricotta cheese
Lunch:
Mixed Vegetable Salad, 8 spears fresh steamed asparagus, baked potato with 1 pat butter. If you're lunching out, order an extra large tossed salad or a chef's salad *without the meat and eggs.*
Dinner:
Spinach Salad (recipe in Chapter 12)
1 cup steamed yellow squash
½ avocado.

Night thought

If you want to accomplish a goal, no matter what it is, you must pay the price!
—ROBERT GORDON COLLIER

DAY FOURTEEN

Headset

This morning, begin to think ahead. On the day after tomorrow, you'll begin a two-day rest from food. The first day you'll fast and the next you'll have only juice. Start now to get your mind set. The mental picture you have of yourself is improving by leaps and bounds! You're truly becoming that image, as you enjoy the simple, live foods you're eating. In your Born-Again journal, describe how you're thinking of yourself today.

Exercise

Sex is a wonderful, fulfilling and motivating force in life. It's also a natural form of exercise. It tones up parts of you that are seldom used in any other activity. Your heart beats faster, increasing from seventy-two beats a minute to three beats a second. Muscles in the buttocks, stomach, and inner thighs become coordinated and active. Breathing and circulation accelerate to a rapid pace. After orgasm, relaxation, tranquility, and a special radiance permeate your entire being. The improvement in your general health and attractiveness—your Born-Again body—will afford you greater opportunity to indulge in this beautiful form of exercise. Think on this as you proceed with the Head-to-Toe exercise regime.

Get out your journal and enter your current measurements alongside those of Days One and Seven. See the improvement!

Food Plan

Choose today's menu from those in Chapter 14.

Night thought

> If a Man (or woman) does not keep pace with his companions, perhaps it is because he (or she) hears a different drummer.
>
> —HENRY DAVID THOREAU

DAY FIFTEEN

Headset

Write down in your notebook: "Tomorrow I will fast. The day after that I will have only juice." Remember to treat yourself as if you were a celebrity. Dinah Shore keeps fantastically young and vibrant by exercising and eating only moderately. She also sets aside one day a week to have only juice and water. This is something you should do when the 30-day plan is over.

Exercise

Go through your entire regime, adding more repetitions. Let today be one of the four times a week (daily is better!) that you run.

Natural grooming tip

Yogurt Facial: After washing and patting dry your face, apply plain yogurt to forehead, cheeks, nose, chin, and neck. Allow the yogurt to remain for 15 minutes (if you work, you can use this time to take your morning bath and organize your outfit for the day).

Remove yogurt with a tissue and rinse off residue with warm water. Pat your face and neck dry with a soft towel. For a nice touch, smooth on some cold pressed oil.

Food Plan

Breakfast:
  2 pears, 6 soaked dried figs
Lunch:
  Large Spinach Salad, steamed green beans, 2 slices whole-grain bread with ½ pat of butter on each slice
Dinner:
  Super Sprouts (recipe in Chapter 13), 1 cup Lentil Stew, Cauliflower Special, 1 cup steamed baby peas
Snack:
  Medium-sized ripe mango or large bunch of black or Ribier grapes.

Night thought

Freedom is the key to beauty. When you have grown to the point where clothes and make-up are no longer ways to hide yourself, and you can accept the way you are, you are free to be beautiful.

—DIANE VON FURSTENBERG
—*Vogue*

DAY SIXTEEN

Headset

Wherever you are, whenever you feel that you're losing your ability to cope, just take a little time out to become mindful of your breathing. You needn't try to alter it. Just become gently *aware* of it. Try it for a few minutes this morning, before you get out of bed.

Exercise

Today, give yourself a total rest, physically as well as physiologically. Skip your calisthenics. Later in the day, take a short walk, just to keep limber.

Natural grooming tip

Get in the habit of reading soap, lotion, and cosmetic labels just as you do food labels. It will surprise you to discover the large amount of chemicals, dyes, perfumes, and potential irritants most of these products contain. Today, buy yourself some pure, untreated soap at a health food store. I suggest Tom's Natural Soap, Argimiel, Lelord Kordel's Special Soap, or a castille soap.

Food Plan

Today is a fasting day. Drink only distilled or spring water.

Night thought

You've successfully resisted temptation and have completed your special day of fasting. Before you go to sleep, think to yourself, "I am forming a lifelong health-giving habit. I feel clean, light, and totally in command of my own body. I'm becoming healthier and more beautiful with each day of my new plan."

> The first wealth is health.
> —RALPH WALDO EMERSON

DAY SEVENTEEN

Headset

As you wake to another day of your new life, reflect on yesterday's foodless day. Fasting becomes easier the more often you do it. This morning you should feel marvelous, mentally as well as physically. Write down in your journal how the fasting feels to you this time, as compared to two weeks ago. You are using your Born-Again journal to develop *awareness* about who you are and how you feel, day in and day out.

Exercise

Since you haven't yet broken your fast, dispense with your calisthenics this morning. Later, after you've had your juice, do some stretching and bending and go for a good, brisk walk.

Natural grooming tip

A good natural toothpaste to use is Tom's, a brand that's available in health food stores. It has no sugar, sweeteners, colorings, abrasives, or preservatives. More and more dentists are beginning to recommend non-abrasive toothpastes, as they've discovered that abrasives and chemicals found in most toothpastes on the market will, over the years, cause erosion of the tooth enamel, especially at the base of the gumline.

Food Plan

Breakfast:
6 ounces fresh orange juice
Midmorning:
6 ounces Green Goddess drink (see recipe p. 112)
Lunch:
6 ounces Pineapple Perfection
Midafternoon:
6 ounces grapefruit juice
Dinner:
Put 2 ripe tomatoes and 2 stalks celery in blender, on high, for 1 minute. Sip slowly or eat with a soupspoon.

Note: Take a thermos of Pineapple Perfection to the office for lunch, if you work. Order your midmorning and afternoon juices *fresh squeezed* (canned or frozen won't do) from a coffee shop. Order any fresh-squeezed juice or juicy piece of melon for lunch if you must eat in a restaurant today.

Night thought

As you stretch out between your nice, crisp sheets, think about the wonderful changes that are taking place within you. It's a sensational, refreshing feeling to know that you're able to be in control of your own life!

> To change, to begin again, is not to deny oneself but to transcend oneself.
>
> —MARTIN GRAY

DAY EIGHTEEN

Headset

Here is a technique that will create greater definition of facial features and bring special radiance to your skin. You can do it before you even sit up this morning.

Open your mouth as wide as you possibly can. Raise your eyebrows way up on your forehead. With mouth open, take the largest inhale you can, making sure to expand both diaphragm and chest.

Hold your breath for five seconds. Then quickly scrunch up your face into a prune. Force everything toward your lips, which you should extend as far forward as possible in an exaggerated kissing pucker. Simultaneously, exhale forcefully through your nostrils.

Breathe normally a few times and repeat. After a session of doing this rapidly, relax while gently massaging your face by moving your open palms in small circles.

Exercise

Weigh in. (You should have lost another pound or two.)

Today, see if you can *double* the number of repetitions Yvonne suggests for each of her exercises. If it's too difficult, don't strain; increase it as much as you're able beyond what you've *been* doing.

Food Plan

Choose your menu today from those in Chapter 14.

Night thought

Today you are sowing the seeds of tomorrow.
What harvest will you reap?
—RAYMOND HULL

DAY NINETEEN

Headset

Begin to prepare for how you're going to live when the 30-day program is over. Put the following notations in your journal: "At times I'll be tempted to overeat, use food as a tranquilizer, lose control or eat wrong foods. I will strive not to let these things happen, but when they do, I won't feel guilty. I will enjoy my deviation and then, rationally, I'll begin all over again."

Exercise

Follow the full exercise program, again, pushing yourself to add to what you did yesterday. Run a mile today or jump rope 3 to 4 minutes.

Natural grooming tip

You'll find that your body odors will naturally become milder as you:

» Clean out some of the debris from your system by fasting.
» Release toxic carbon dioxide through vigorous breathing from jogging and jumping rope.
» Cut out the kinds of food and chemicals that leave a garbage residue in your cells.
» Increase the amounts of chlorophyl foods—raw, green, leafy vegetables—in your diet.

Food Plan

Today's menu:

Breakfast:
Large bowl of fresh unsweetened blueberries and strawberries with ½ cup light cream and 1 tbsp. sunflower seeds
Lunch:
Large tossed salad if you eat out, celery, small tomatoes and cucumber sticks if you take lunch to the office. Half an avocado or ½ cup cottage cheese, 1 cup steamed broccoli or any steamed vegetable if you eat at home.
Dinner:
Plain Finger salad (no dressing)
1 cup steamed green lima beans
1 baked potato with pat of butter
Snack:
1 pear

Night thought

As you relax into the restorative phase of your daily cycle, remind yourself that success lies not in never falling, but in picking yourself right back up when you do.

Never say die, say damn!
—OLD SAYING

DAY TWENTY

Headset

This morning, increase your chances for the long-term success of your new life by affirming the powerful law of cause and effect. Take out your notebook and enter these words: "When I *choose* to practice positive eating and living habits, I am really choosing to be vibrant, youthful, and thin. Recognizing the existence of this immutable law of cause and effect will help take the randomness out of life and myself."

Exercise

Today go through the Head-to-Toe Shape-Up Plan. Raise the number of repetitions of exercises 8, 10, 12, 16 and 18 to *three times* the amount given.

Food Plan

Choose your menu plan for today from the menu chapter. Put thought into making your salad as appealing as possible: a variety of fresh, crispy greens and firm, colorful vegetables, served in a pretty bowl and set out on your prettiest place mat.

Night thought

As you relax into sleep, congratulate yourself for mastering this new, disciplined approach to health. You're looking better and feeling better. Best of all, you know it's no fluke but the result of care and effort on your part.

Let each man (or woman) become all that he (she) was created capable of being.
—THOMAS CARLYLE

DAY TWENTY-ONE

Headset

Today is a day to renew motivation. Note the following in your journal: "If I want permanent changes in my health . . . if I want to stay younger longer . . . if I want to be vibrant, sexy, active, and beautiful . . . if I want to avoid chronic diseases of old age . . . *I must be willing to make the principles I'm learning a permanent part of my life.*

Exercise

Today, raise the number of repetitions of exercises 9, 11, 13, 15 and 17 to *three times* the amount given. In addition, spend 5 minutes jumping rope (you can do this later in the day) *or* running a mile and a quarter.

Food Plan

To break up the strict routine you're on, invite some friends for lunch or dinner tomorrow. Start preparing today. Plan to serve whole-wheat lasagna, a large salad, green peas, and crudités.
Today's menu:

Breakfast:
1 whole papaya, large bunch white grapes
Lunch:
Pineapple Delight
Dinner:
Fresh Green Pea Soup
Buttercrunch Salad
1 cup steamed brown rice, small pat butter
1 cup steamed carrots
Snack:
2 large nectarines

Night thought

Accept any "catches" or discordant notes that may have occurred today. (Some people call them mistakes but I prefer to think of them as learning experiences.) Weave them into the pattern of your thought blanket. Its texture will be enriched by the contrast.

Failure can be instructive.
—WAYNE W. DYER

DAY TWENTY-TWO
Headset

Here's a mental exercise that will empty you of any distressing or frenzied thoughts that may be crowding you this morning. You should do it before rising.

Your hand should be resting comfortably, palm up, on the bed. With your eyes closed, just think about your hand for a minute. Try to feel all the muscles and sinews and bones: try to feel the weight of the atmosphere on the skin of your palm. As you think about your hand, become aware also of your breathing. In comes the good air—out goes the bad air.

Now, from the flat-palm-upward position, slowly, ever so slowly, begin to curl your thumb and forefinger toward each other (remember, eyes closed for this). The trick here is to do it *slowly,* as slowly as you possibly can while still moving. You want to curl both thumb and finger around until they make a closed circle and the tips should touch *as lightly as possible.*

After you've touched thumb and forefinger, slowly return them to their original positions. Now do the same thing with each of your fingers in succession. After finishing one hand, move on to the other.

When you've finished slow hand meditation with both hands, inhale and exhale deeply, and gently lift your eyelids. Calmer?

Exercise

John, a stylist at Saks Fifth Avenue's beauty salon, shared with me this excellent stomach flattener.

» *Lie on your back on the floor. Keeping your legs straight and toes pointed, raise your legs about six inches off the floor.*
» *With the toes of your right foot, begin forming the letters of the alphabet in the air, breathing in through your nostrils on one stroke of the letter, out through your mouth on the next. Draw the next letter with the toes of your left foot and alternate back and forth with each letter.*

» *The first day, take six letters. Add a letter a day until you've completed the alphabet in one session.*

Substitute this exercise for the sit-ups in Yvonne's exercise plan one day a week. You'll know it's working by the temporary soreness in your stomach muscles.

Food Plan

Today you have a luncheon or dinner to enjoy with your friends. If it's lunch, skip dinner tonight to make up for your larger lunch, or make it a light dinner: a refreshing citrus fruit salad or a plate of sliced melon. If it's dinner, skip lunch.

Choose your remaining meals from the menus in Chapter 14.

Night thought

Before giving yourself over, tonight, to nature's miraculous repair forces, rejoice in the new-found truths that are leading you into a fresh new life of health and happiness.

Viewed in any and all aspects, Health is Life.
—HERBERT M. SHELTON

DAY TWENTY-THREE

Headset

Accept the fact that, as it took time for your health problems to evolve, it will also take time to halt and reverse those abnormal changes. The self-discipline you're exerting will help to erase the errors you've made in the past. List in your notebook all the positive changes you've instituted so far. Compare it with the list of goals you made on Day Six. Is there something you're avoiding? Commit yourself to face up to it.

Natural grooming tip

If you have a problem with dry hair, don't shampoo it for a week. Brush your hair every day with a natural-bristle brush, distributing the oils throughout your hair. At the end of the week, shampoo, rinse, and see how much softer your crowning glory is! Do this until your hair is in better shape.

Exercise

Look yourself over in the mirror this morning. Notice the overall improvement in your figure, skin tone, hair, eyes. Take your measurements and compare them to those of Day One. Let your pride inspire you to continue the morning Shape-Up workouts with renewed vigor.

Food Plan

Breakfast:
½ fresh pineapple, 1 ounce raw pumpkin seeds
Lunch:
Fresh Fruit Special
Dinner:
Mixed green salad, 1 ear fresh corn, steamed escarole, baked potato, 1 pat butter

Night thought

The laws of chemistry act as unswervingly in the human body as they do in the chemical laboratory.
—SCOTT NEARING

DAY TWENTY-FOUR

Headset

During your think-time this morning, give a special thought to the role discipline plays in the new life you're creating for yourself. Discipline is often given a negative connotation but in fact it means "to learn," and learning is an adventure, an exciting challenge. Begin to think of *your* discipline as an exciting learning experience.

Exercise

As you go through your morning routine, with mirror and exercise, think about how much sexier you've become since you've started your Born-Again Body Program. Sex is a wonderful pleasure. Direct more energy into this joyous part of your life. Here's a special sexercise you can practice anytime, anywhere: Alternately tense and relax your vaginal muscles. See how hard you can squeeze—relax—squeeze—relax. Repeat 10 times. Practice several times a day—as you drive, as you type, as you prepare your family's meals. Your husband or lover will adore your practicing it on him!

Today, take a vacation from the Head-to-Toe Exercise regimen.

Natural grooming tip

For a natural facial, rub avocado peel over your face and leave it on 5 or 6 minutes before rinsing off with warm water. The natural oils will make your skin feel soft and smooth.

Food Plan

Select from the menus in Chapter 14.

Night thought

> All the progress the world has ever made has been by breaking with tradition, branching out into new and untrodden fields.
>
> —HERBERT SHELTON

DAY TWENTY-FIVE

Headset

Learn to free your own mind, think for yourself, live for yourself. Vested interests control the minds of the overwhelming majority of your fellow travelers in life. You must develop the strength to do your own thinking, to choose for yourself the simple, uncomplicated way of life that brings health and longevity. For help with this, read books like *Walden* by Henry David Thoreau, *Nature* by Ralph Waldo Emerson, *The Dragons of Eden* by Carl Sagan, *Animal Liberation* by Peter Singer, and *Health for the Millions* by Herbert M. Shelton.

Exercise

This morning, lie face down on the floor and try out this new stomach-control exercise. With your arms stretched straight out in front of you, legs straight behind you and slightly apart, lift your chest off the floor. At the same time, lift your still-straight arms and legs as far off the floor as you can. Lift, relax; lift, relax. Repeat 10 times (if you can).

Go through Exercises 1 through 20 *twice,* from beginning to end.

Food Plan

Breakfast:
  Tropical Treat
            or
  3 ripe peaches
Lunch:
  Bowl of hot vegetable soup (2 cups)
  3 stalks crisp green celery
Dinner:
  Sunburst Salad
  1 cup green peas, lightly steamed
  Stuffed Eggplant

Night thought

Your 30-Day Program is almost over. This brings up some uneasy feelings. You've got a decision ahead of you. After the month is up, there are two ways you can go. You can resume the hit-or-miss way you were living a month ago, following your whims, letting the media and the rest of society determine your lifestyle. *Or,* you can opt for the new way, the dynamic, health-giving, excitingly high-energy way you've been learning about these past weeks.

> Stretch out your hand and grasp the plus, which, maybe, you have never made use of, save in great emergencies. LIFE IS AN EMERGENCY MOST GRAVE.
> —FREDERICK VAN RENSSELAER DEY

DAY TWENTY-SIX

Headset

Imagine yourself in all your glory: slim, healthy, youthful, vibrant—just as you'd like to be. Through following the 30-Day Program you're approaching that goal. You've done your fasting and exercising, you've followed the food plan and have learned how to control your daily actions by communicating with your inner self each morning. To keep the new, "I-care-about-me" attitude you've developed, decide *now* to make your new habits permanent ones.

Today, write in your journal whatever random thoughts come to mind. Just let loose, no holds barred. You might surprise yourself.

Exercise

Go through your daily session at the mirror, beginning with exercise 1 and going through to 20. These are now *your* exercises. Never give them up. Today, pick three spots that still need special work and do extra repetitions of those exercises. Do one of the relaxing exercises between each set of extra repetitions.

Natural grooming tip

Peel half a cucumber, cut it into chunks, and blend on high for a few seconds. Pat this mixture on your face, let it soak into your pores, and then rinse with tepid water. Cucumber is a natural astringent. This masque will make your skin feel fresh and tingly.

Food Plan

Choose your menu today from those in Chapter 14.

Night thought

Be thankful, tonight, for your new self-awareness. Affirm that you will never lose sight of who you are; that you'll never forget your capacity for joy, for doing and for being a dynamic, fulfilled human being.

> Be who you are and become all you were meant to be, which is the only winning game in the world.
> —SIDNEY J. HARRIS

DAY TWENTY-SEVEN

Headset

Today, take those measurements again. Jot them down in your notebook. They should inspire you the next time you decide to go on a mini-fast.

Exercise

Do your regular exercises today. Time yourself. Do as many extra repetitions as *you* think necessary. Commit yourself to this amount of time for working out *every day* (or almost) of your life!

Natural grooming tip

Don't use a rinse after your next shampoo. You'll find, as I have, that your hair actually feels cleaner and has more body when you *don't* use one of those expensive commercial "conditioners."

Food Plan

Breakfast:
Large slice of watermelon
Lunch:
1 large banana, ½ cup raisins, 2 pears
Dinner:
Large Finger Salad, 2 large juicy ripe tomatoes, ½ cup pecan halves
Snack:
1 cup of fresh sweet cherries

Night thought

As you add your finishing thoughts to this day, remind yourself that health and beauty are not just haphazard states that you fall into if you're lucky. It takes knowledge, awareness, and a special strength for most of us to acquire them. If we want good health and golden good looks we must choose and then earn them.

> There is something beautiful about most women, but often they don't know it.
> —FRANCESCO SCAVULLO

DAY TWENTY-EIGHT

Headset

This morning, decide to live. Do this and you will, by the plan set out for you in this book:
1) maintain your sense of self-respect and self-importance
2) live with less pain, both mentally and physically
3) cope adequately with your daily living from now on.

Exercise

Face yourself in the mirror. Notice the deliciously invigorating change that's taking place, outside as well as inside your body.

If you can do it without strain, do the Head-to-Toe regimen three times today, just to show yourself how much *stronger* you've gotten.

Natural grooming tip

The best skin tonic is a clean and healthy bloodstream. All the lotions, creams, and preparations you may use are minor in usefulness compared to the nourishment your skin gets when fed by clean, healthy blood. Remember to think green, and to include generous amounts of leafy and other greens in your daily diet. Make yourself a Green Goddess drink today! (See recipe on p. 112.)

Food Plan

Choose your meals for today from Chapter 14.

Night thought

Never forget that there are two of you: the positive you and the negative you. You can choose either personality as the dominant one in your life. Think, tonight, about all the beautiful aspects of the positive you. Say to yourself, "I will continue to develop the beautiful, positive me!"

To become or not to become—That is the question.
—Floyd W. Matson

DAY TWENTY-NINE

Headset

Your 30 days are almost completed. Just think! This is the twenty-ninth morning you've quietly put your thoughts in order and programmed yourself for a productive day. Get out the journal you've been keeping during this period. Make a list of the improvements you've wrought, physically and mentally, since Day One. If *your* notebook compares with mine (I've fasted and gone on the regime, too) you'll be anywhere from five to twenty pounds lighter, eyes sparkling—aches and pains diminished. Your energy for life is way up.

Exercise

With one more day to go in the 30-Day Program, congratulate yourself for having stuck with your exercises every day for a month. Pride in your new contours and a new feeling of aliveness makes your previous days' struggle to remain active worthwhile. You've proved to yourself that exercising needn't be dreadful, but can be invigorating and energy-raising. Put extra zip into your daily dozen this morning!

Food Plan

Follow a Mono-meal plan today. An extra pound or two lost will set an even prouder tone on which to end your Born-Again Program.

Breakfast:
A whole melon of your choice—honeydew, cantaloupe, casaba, or Spanish, or a large piece of watermelon
Midmorning:
Green Goddess drink
Lunch:
Several bunches of your favorite kind of grapes
Dinner:
Large vegetable salad

Night thought

You feel marvelous—relaxed and in control. As you prepare your mind and body for rest on this next-to-last evening of your

30-Day Program, be quietly, joyously proud of *you*. Your life has taken on a newness and freshness that defies description. Decide to keep it this way.

> If you are going to be born again, what matters is how you live today, because today is going to sow the seed of beauty—or the seed of sorrow.
>
> —J. KRISHNAMURTI

DAY THIRTY

Headset

This is the final day of your Born-Again Body Program. Set your mind and total self for the specialness of the day! Decide to wear something especially becoming. Decide to celebrate. Go out to dinner or even take a special vacation if you're able. You've gone through the entire 30 days and you are TERRIFIC!

Exercise

This is Celebration Day. Do a quick run-through with Yvonne (exercises 1 through 20 *once*) and then get outside and run your joyous route. Let the beautiful awareness of life take over as the fresh air fills your lungs and the sun and gentle winds play on your skin. Remind yourself, for this Day of Celebration and for all future days, that Life is Activity. Plan to get more of it into your daily life.

Natural grooming tip

True beauty comes from within. A healthy, well-functioning body is reflected outward in the form of glowing skin, sparkling eyes, shiny hair and a happy disposition. By now you have them all!

Food Plan

Have your breakfast and lunch today from my menus. You now appreciate the fine, satisfying flavors of the sun-cooked fresh foods you've been eating. You feel fresher and cleaner inside and out. Fringe benefits of this eating plan are: 1) your teeth have a clean feel, 2) your catarrhal condition has cleared up, and 3) your bowel habits have improved. Now, you're on your own. Choose wisely and know, for all future time, the benefits to be derived from a diet predominant in live foods.

Enjoy dinner out this evening. Let it be a celebration of your 30-day accomplishment!

Night thought

You've learned that communicating with yourself at the beginning and at the end of each day is a rewarding habit that helps you find peace of mind, self-awareness, and self-control. Continue to put aside time for your Headset and Night thought as you strive to live the Born-Again life.

> Dream lofty dreams, and as you dream, so shall you become. Your vision is the promise of what you shall one day be. Your ideal is the prophecy of what you shall at last unveil.
>
> —James Allen

THE QUESTIONS I'M ASKED MOST FREQUENTLY

CHAPTER 22

Frequently Asked Questions

Q. *With so much emphasis on dieting and weight loss during recent years hasn't the average American become thinner and healthier?*

A. Would that it were so, but the answer is no. Believe it or not, American men and women are *more* overweight than they were a decade ago. A survey by the National Center for Health Statistics shows that the average American male weighs twenty to thirty pounds more than he ought to, and four pounds more than he did ten years before the survey was conducted, in 1974. The average woman weighs fifteen to thirty pounds too much, and a pound more than she did in 1964.

Q. *Why is this happening, in spite of the apparent increase in health awareness of so many people?*

A. The problem lies in the rise of the fast-food industry and the growing popularity of junk food, says Sydney Abraham, chief of the above-mentioned statistics center. These non-foods create malnutrition with its concomitant fluid retention and fat accumulation.

Q. *What's the difference between the fad diets that have come and gone through the years—things like the "grapefruit diet," the "high-protein diets," the "drinking man's diet"—and the new way of eating you describe in this book?*

A. Fad diets are lopsided, unbalanced approaches to weight loss that are definitely unhealthy, especially when followed over a long period of time. The best way to lose weight, improve your health, and keep thin, is to permanently switch to a well-balanced, *healthy* way of eating such as the New Lifetime Eating Plan described in this book.

Q. *I've heard the so-called "protein-sparing" diet can be dangerous. Why is this so?*

A. Medical experts say it creates an electrolyte imbalance in the body that can interfere with the proper functioning of the heart, liver, kidneys, and pancreas. If persisted in, such a diet may result in hepatitis, nephritis, and even heart stoppage.

Q. *If you want to lose weight, isn't it better to diet sensibly than to fast?*

A. While a sensible, healthful way of eating is essential for losing weight properly, I agree with Dr. Walter Bloom, of Piedmont Hospital in Atlanta, Georgia, who stated in the *Journal of the American Medical Association* that fasting is easier on the body than going suddenly from a large food intake to a small one.

Q. *What are the main advantages of fasting?*

A. Fasting cleanses, purifies, and desalinates your entire system. It removes *the causes* of fluid retention and fat accumulation, cleanses the taste buds of the tongue, and normalizes the gastro-intestinal tract. As for helping you change your way of eating, fasting breaks up reflex habit-patterns and paves the way for healthy eating. Last, but far from least, fasting re-energizes.

Q. *I have heard that fasting is dangerous because it uses up lean muscle tissue. Is this true?*

A. You'd have to fast for a very long time for this to start happening. The body doesn't begin consuming its own lean muscle tissue until it has entered the clinical state of starvation. If you were to fast on your own for three or four days, you'd never come close to starvation. If you were to go away to a fasting institution for a longer period of time, you'd be under the supervision of a competent practitioner, who has various methods of determining when a fast should be broken, including measuring the level of urea and nitrogen in the blood.

Q. *Are there people who shouldn't fast at all?*

A. Yes. Those without any knowledge of fasting shouldn't try it. You need to understand some things about the basic physiology of fasting and also that there are precautions to take under certain circumstances. You will have the basic information you need for a short fast if you read Chapter 7 in this book. However, if you're on certain types of medication such as digitalis, cortisone, dicumerol, mezantone, insulin, and some types of thyroid medications, *you should fast only under competent supervision.*

Q. *How much weight will I lose while fasting, and how quickly?*

A. Everyone's metabolism is different, so it's impossible to make guarantees, but generally, taller people lose more in a given time than shorter ones. The average faster will lose about two pounds a day for the first five days; after that, the rate of loss diminishes somewhat.

Q. *What are the arguments in favor of vegetarianism?*

A. Vegetarianism used to be considered kooky or cultish. Today more and more people are becoming vegetarians, and the arguments in favor of it are coming from stronger and stronger sources. Some of the main reasons to stop eating meat, poultry, and fish are:

1) *Better health.* Dr. David Rush, associate professor of public health and member of the Institute of Human Nutrition at Columbia University, says vegetarians who eat well-balanced meals are well nourished. "On the average, vegetarians seem far healthier than others—they are leaner, and have strikingly lower blood pressure and serum cholesterol levels. Many doctors also believe the vegetarian diet reduces one's chances of getting diverticulitis, appendicitis, and cancer of the intestine."

2) *Less heart disease.* The Inter-Society Commission for Heart Disease Resources, established by the government to study coronary disease, has advised Americans to limit their intake of meat and increase their consumption of grains, fruits, vegetables, and legumes of all kinds.

3) *Less cancer.* A sizzling charcoal-broiled steak may smell tempting, but it may carry (per pound) as much benzopyrene (a known cancer-stimulating agent) as the smoke of 300 cigarettes. Even cooking meat at high temperature leads to the production of methycholanthrene, a toxic chemical that has caused cancer in lab animals.

"Cancer can also be transferred directly in the meat itself. When cancer is found in animals," writes Dr. John A. Schaffffenberg, associate professor of nutrition at the School of Health at Loma Linda University, in California, "it is removed; but the rest of the carcass is usually passed for food. The removal of a tumor does not necessarily remove all cancerous cells. The blood or lymphatic system may have already spread such cells to other parts of the body."

4) *Ample protein and lower caloric and fat intake.* In 1973 the Food and Nutrition Board of the National Research Council in Washington, D.C., reported that both lacto-ovovegetarians and total vegetarians had more than enough protein. In fact, most Americans eat at least twice the amount of protein they need, and excess protein turns to fat. Much of the fat in the American diet is contained in meats. These fats make the calorie count of even the so-called "lean" meats zoom. Natural carbohydrates—fruits, vegetables, and whole or unprocessed grains—are low in calories and fats.

5) *The metabolism of meat or animal protein has an aging effect on the human body.* Animal protein is very complex stuff that needs to be broken down and then reconstituted before the body can use it at all. In the process, toxic by-products of the breakdown, urea and uric acid, are thrown into the bloodstream and need to be gotten rid of by the liver and kidneys. All this unnecessary work on the part of the body's internal organs ages it prematurely. Plant protein metabolism is much easier on the body. Carbohydrate metabolism is easier still.

Q. *Don't you get more chemical pesticides from eating fruit and vegetables than from eating meat?*

A. No. Animals that feed on chemically treated hay and vegetation store those poisons in their tissues. The concentration of toxic residue is far greater in flesh foods than in produce—not to mention the harmful hormones, dyes, and preservatives so heavily relied on in modern meat-packaging methods.

Q. *Do vegetarians eat cheese and eggs?*

A. Vegetarians who include cheese and eggs in their diets are called lacto-ovo vegetarians.

Q. *Is milk a good food for adults?*

A. No. Once animals—including humans—reach the weaning stage, milk is no longer needed, nor is it usually well tolerated. Lactase, the enzyme that digests milk, disappears from the human digestive tract after infancy. Renin, the gastric enzyme that coagulates milk, disappears completely by the time the child is seven. Pediatricians and nutritionists now recognize that many allergies and diseases of childhood and adulthood can be traced to overconsumption of milk in early life and after.

Q. *What about cheese? It's a milk product.*
A. Cheese is somewhat easier to handle than milk since it's already been predigested by the addition of renet.

Q. *What about yogurt?*
A. Yogurt is made by adding a bacterial culture, acidophilus, to milk. This is another method of predigestion. Unsweetened plain yogurt is all right, but it's not the magic health food you may have been led by the dairy industry to believe that it is. Also, many commercial yogurts have chemical preservatives and "fillers" added. Check the labels carefully.

Q. *Do you use vitamin supplements as a part of your diet?*
A. No, I don't, and I never have. Neither have any of my family. Vitamins and minerals are supplied best by a good diet and can't be duplicated by a chemist. Nutritionists are beginning to warn of the dangers of hypervitaminosis. The American Medical Association says overuse of vitamins is on the verge of becoming a major health problem in the United States.

Q. *What foods do you rely on for protein?*
A. Dark, green leafy vegetables such as romaine lettuce, kale, and parsley are high in amino acid content. I eat these in large quantity. In lesser quantity I eat nuts and natural nut butters, avocado, lentils, potatoes, and sprouts. I also eat natural cheeses such as cottage, ricotta, and muenster in moderation.

Q. *What are some good, fast-energy carbohydrate foods?*
A. Ripe oranges, melons (especially watermelon), grapes, bananas, figs, raisins, and dates. These and other naturally occurring fruit sugars are easy to assimilate and are well balanced with minerals, vitamins, natural juices, sugars, and fiber. *They produce more energy with less expenditure in return than any other food you can eat.*

APPENDIX A

RECOMMENDED FASTING RETREATS

Bay 'N Gulf Health Resort
18207-09 Gulf Blvd.
Redington Shores
St. Petersburg, Florida 33708
(813) 392-8326

Dr. Shelton's Health School
P. O. Box 1277
San Antonio, Texas 78295
(512) 438-2454

Esser's Hygienic Rest Ranch
P.O. Box 161
Lake Worth, Florida
(305) 965-4360

"Kawana"
Cobah Road
Arcadia, 2159, Australia

Pawling Health Manor
P.O. Box 401
Hyde Park, New York 12538
(914) 889-4141

Scott's Natural Health Institute
P.O. Box 8919
Cleveland, Ohio 44136
(216) 238-6930

Shalimar Health Home
First Avenue
Frinton-On-Sea
Essex, England

VACATION RETREATS

Shangri-La Natural Hygiene
  Institute
Bonita Springs, Florida 33923
(813) 992-3811

Sun Crest Educational Resort
Box H, 501 Old Harding Highway
Malaga, New Jersey 08328
(609) 694-2887

Villa Vegetariana Health Resort
P.O. Box 1228
Cuernavaca, Morelos, Mexico

WEST COAST CONSULTANTS

Gerald Benesh, D.C.
1450 West Mission Road
San Marcos, California 92069
(714) 744-0118

Ralph C. Cinque, D.C.
15300 Ventura Blvd.
Sherman Oaks, California 91403
(312) 986-7163

APPENDIX B

MAIL ORDER SOURCES FOR FRUITS, VEGETABLES AND NUTS

CALIFORNIA

Covalda Date Co.   Dried Fruit and Nuts
P.O. Box 908
Coachella, 92236

Jaffe Brothers   Dried Fruit and Nuts
28560 Lilac Road
Valley Center 92082

FLORIDA

Orange Grove Health Ranch   Organically grown citrus
Box 316, Route 4
Arcadia 32821-R

Lee's Fruit Company   Citrus, November through June
Leesburg

All Organics, Inc.   Avocados, July through March
15870 S.W. 216th St.   Mangoes, July through September
Miami 33170   Citrus, November through June

Axel T. Peterson   Organically grown citrus
Vero Beach

APPENDIX C

Portion	Calories	Protein Grams	Fat	Carbo-hydrates Grams
DAIRY PRODUCTS				
Cheese, natural				
Blue or Roquefort type, 1 oz	100	6	8	1
Camembert, $\frac{1}{3}$ of 4 oz container	115	8	9	Trace
Cheddar, 1 oz	115	7	9	Trace
Shredded, 1 cup	455	28	37	1
Cottage				
Creamed, 1 cup	235	28	10	6
Low fat, 1 cup	205	31	4	8
Dry curd, 1 cup	125	25	1	3
Cream, 1 oz	100	2	10	1
Mozzarella, whole milk, 1 oz	90	6	7	1
Parmesan, grated, 1 tbsp	25	2	2	Trace
Provolone, 1 oz	100	7	8	1
Ricotta, 1 cup	428	28	32	7
Romano, 1 oz	110	9	8	1
Swiss, 1 oz	105	8	8	1
Cheese, pasteurized process				
American, 1 oz	105	6	9	Trace
Spread, American, 1 oz	82	5	6	2
Cream, sweet				
Half-and-half				
1 cup	315	7	28	10
1 tbsp	20	Trace	2	1
Light, coffee or table				
1 cup	470	6	46	9
1 tbsp	30	Trace	3	1
Whipping, before whipping				
1 cup	820	5	88	7
1 tbsp	80	Trace	6	Trace
Whipped topping, 1 tbsp	10	Trace	1	Trace
Cream, sour				
1 cup	495	7	48	10
1 tbsp	25	Trace	3	1
Cream products, imitation				
Sweet:				
Creamers				
Liquid (frozen), 1 tbsp	20	Trace	1	2
Powdered, 1 tbsp	10	Trace	1	1

Portion	Calories	Protein Grams	Fat	Carbo-hydrates Grams
Creamed products, imitation (Cont'd):				
Sweet (Cont'd):				
Whipped topping				
Frozen, 1 tbsp	15	Trace	1	1
Pressurized, 1 tbsp	10	Trace	1	1
Imitation sour cream				
1 cup	415	8	39	11
1 tbsp	20	Trace	2	1
Milk				
Whole, 1 cup	150	8	8	11
Lowfat, 1 cup	120	8	5	12
Nonfat (skim), 1 cup	85	8	Trace	12
Buttermilk, 1 cup	100	8	2	12
Canned, evaporated, 1 cup	340	17	19	25
Dried, nonfat instant				
1 envelope	325	32	1	47
1 cup	245	24	Trace	35
Milk beverages				
Chocolate milk, 1 cup	210	8	8	26
Milk desserts, frozen				
Ice cream				
Regular (about 11% fat)				
$\frac{1}{2}$ gal	2,155	38	115	254
1 cup	270	5	14	32
3 fl oz	100	2	5	12
Soft serve (frozen custard), 1 cup	375	7	23	38
Ice milk, hardened (about 4.3% fat)				
$\frac{1}{2}$ gal	1,470	41	45	232
1 cup	185	5	6	29
Sherbet (about 2% fat)				
$\frac{1}{2}$ gal	2,160	17	31	469
1 cup	270	2	4	59
Yogurt:				
Made with lowfat milk:				
Fruit flavored, 1 8-oz container	230	10	3	42
Plain, 1 8-oz container	145	12	4	16
Made with whole milk, 1 8-oz container	140	8	7	11

EGGS

Portion	Calories	Protein Grams	Fat	Carbo-hydrates Grams
Eggs, large (24 oz per dozen), 1 egg	80	6	6	1

FATS, OILS: RELATED PRODUCTS

Portion	Calories	Protein Grams	Fat	Carbo-hydrates Grams
Butter				
Regular				
1 $\frac{1}{4}$-lb stick ($\frac{1}{2}$ cup)	815	1	92	Trace
1 tbsp	100	Trace	12	Trace
Whipped				
1 $\frac{1}{4}$-lb stick ($\frac{1}{2}$ cup)	540	1	61	Trace
1 tbsp	65	Trace	8	Trace
Margarine, regular				
1 $\frac{1}{4}$-lb stick ($\frac{1}{2}$ cup)	815	1	92	Trace
1 tbsp	100	Trace	12	Trace

Portion	Calories	Protein Grams	Fat	Carbo-hydrates Grams
Oils, salad or cooking				
Corn				
1 cup	1,925	0	218	0
1 tbsp	120	0	14	0
Olive				
1 cup	1,910	0	216	0
1 tbsp	120	0	14	0
Peanut				
1 cup	1,910	0	216	0
1 tbsp	120	0	14	0
Safflower				
1 cup	1,925	0	218	0
1 tbsp	120	0	14	0
Salad dressings				
Commercial				
French				
Regular, 1 tbsp	65	Trace	6	3
Low calorie (5 cal per tsp), 1 tbsp	15	Trace	1	2
Italian				
Regular, 1 tbsp	85	Trace	9	1
Low calorie (2 cal per tsp), 1 tbsp	10	Trace	1	Trace
Mayonnaise, 1 tbsp	100	Trace	11	Trace

FISH, MEAT, POULTRY: RELATED PRODUCTS

Portion	Calories	Protein Grams	Fat	Carbo-hydrates Grams
Fish and shellfish:				
Bluefish, baked with butter or margarine, 3 oz	135	22	4	0
Haddock, breaded, fried, 3 oz	140	17	5	5
Ocean perch, breaded, fried, 1 fillet	195	16	11	6
Salmon, pink, canned, solids and liquid, 3 oz	120	17	5	0
Sardines, Atlantic, canned in oil, drained				
solids, 3 oz	175	20	9	0
Tuna, canned in oil, drained solids, 3 oz	170	24	7	0
Meat and meat products:				
Beef, cooked:				
Cuts braised, simmered or pot roasted:				
Lean and fat (piece, $2\frac{1}{2}$" by $2\frac{1}{2}$" by				
$\frac{3}{4}$"), 3 oz	245	23	16	0
Ground beef, broiled:				
Lean with 10% fat, 3 oz or patty 3" by				
$\frac{5}{8}$"	185	23	5	0
Steak:				
Relatively fat sirloin, broiled:				
Lean and fat (piece $2\frac{1}{2}$" by $2\frac{1}{2}$" by				
$\frac{3}{4}$"), 3 oz	330	20	27	0
Lean only, 2 oz	115	18	4	0
Relatively lean round, braised:				
Lean and fat (piece $4\frac{1}{8}$" by $2\frac{1}{4}$" by				
$\frac{1}{2}$"), 3 oz	220	24	13	0
Lamb, cooked:				
Chop:				
Lean and fat, 3.1 oz	360	18	32	0
Leg, roasted:				
Lean and fat (2 pieces $4\frac{1}{8}$" by $2\frac{1}{4}$" by				
$\frac{1}{4}$"), 3 oz	235	22	16	0

Portion	Calories	Protein Grams	Fat	Carbo-hydrates Grams
Meat and meat products (Cont'd):				
Pork, cured, cooked:				
Ham, light cure, lean and fat, roasted				
(2 pieces, $4\frac{1}{8}$" by $2\frac{1}{4}$" by				
$\frac{1}{4}$"), 3 oz	245	18	19	0
Pork, fresh, cooked:				
Chop, loin (cut 3 per lb with bone), broiled:				
Lean and fat, 2.7 oz	305	19	25	0
Roast, oven cooked, no liquid added:				
Lean and fat (piece $2\frac{1}{2}$" by $2\frac{1}{2}$" by				
$\frac{3}{4}$"), 3 oz	310	21	24	0
Sausages:				
Brown and serve (10–11 per 8-oz pkg),				
browned, 1 link	70	3	6	Trace
Frankfurter (8 per 1-lb pkg), cooked				
(reheated), 1 frankfurter	170	7	15	1
Pork link (16 per 1-lb pkg), cooked,				
1 link	60	2	6	Trace
Veal, medium fat, cooked, bone removed:				
Cutlet ($4\frac{1}{8}$" by $2\frac{1}{4}$" by $\frac{1}{2}$"), braised or				
broiled, 3 oz	185	23	9	0
Poultry and poultry products:				
Chicken, half broiler, broiled, bones removed				
(10.4 oz with bones), 6.2 oz	240	42	7	0
Chicken Chow Mein, canned, 1 cup	95	7	Trace	18
Turkey, roasted, flesh without skin:				
Dark meat, piece $2\frac{1}{2}$" by $1\frac{5}{8}$" by $\frac{1}{4}$",				
4 pieces	175	26	7	0
Light meat, piece, 4" by 2" by $\frac{1}{4}$", 2 pieces	150	28	3	0

FRUITS AND FRUIT PRODUCTS

Portion	Calories	Protein Grams	Fat	Carbo-hydrates Grams
Apples, raw, unpeeled, without cores, $2\frac{3}{4}$" diam.				
(about 3 per lb with cores), 1 apple	80	Trace	1	20
Applejuice, bottled or canned, 1 cup	120	Trace	Trace	30
Apricots:				
Raw, without pits (about 12 per lb with pits),				
3 apricots	55	1	Trace	14
Canned in heavy syrup (halves and syrup), 1 cup	220	2	Trace	57
Dried				
Uncooked (28 large or 37 medium halves per				
cup), 1 cup	340	7	1	86
Cooked, unsweetened, fruit and liquid, 1 cup	215	4	1	54
Avocados, 1 avocado	370	5	37	13
Banana, 1 banana	100	1	Trace	26
Blueberries, raw, 1 cup	90	1	1	22
Cherries				
Sour, canned, 1 cup	105	2	Trace	26
Sweet, raw, 10 cherries	45	1	Trace	12
Cranberry juice cocktail, bottled, sweetened, 1 cup	165	Trace	Trace	42
Cranberry sauce, sweetened, canned, 1 cup	405	Trace	1	104
Dates, 10 dates	220	2	Trace	58
Fruit cocktail, canned, in heavy syrup, 1 cup	195	1	Trace	50
Grapefruit, $\frac{1}{2}$ grapefruit	50	1	Trace	13

Portion	Calories	Protein Grams	Fat	Carbo-hydrates Grams
Grapefruit juice				
Canned				
Unsweetened, 1 cup	100	1	Trace	24
Sweetened, 1 cup	135	1	Trace	32
Frozen, concentrate, unsweetened, undiluted				
6 fl oz can	300	4	1	72
Grapes, raw, 10 grapes	35	Trace	Trace	9
Grape juice, canned or bottled, 1 cup	165	1	Trace	42
Grape drink, canned, 1 cup	135	Trace	Trace	35
Lemonade concentrate, frozen, undiluted,				
6 fl oz can	425	Trace	Trace	112
Melon–Cantaloupe, $\frac{1}{2}$ melon	80	2	Trace	20
Oranges, 1 orange	65	1	Trace	16
Orange juice				
Raw, 1 cup	110	2	Trace	26
Frozen concentrate, undiluted, 6 fl oz can	360	5	Trace	87
Peaches				
Whole, 1 peach	40	1	Trace	10
Canned in syrup pack, 1 cup	200	1	Trace	51
Frozen, 1 cup	220	1	Trace	57
Pears				
Raw, 1 pear	100	1	1	25
Canned in syrup, 1 cup	195	1	1	50
Pineapple				
Raw diced, 1 cup	80	1	Trace	21
Canned in syrup				
Crushed, chunks, tidbits, 1 cup	190	1	Trace	49
Slices and liquid, 1 slice	80	Trace	Trace	20
Pineapple juice, unsweetened, canned, 1 cup	140	1	Trace	34
Plums				
Raw, prune type, 1 plum	20	Trace	Trace	6
Canned, heavy syrup pack, 1 cup	215	1	Trace	56
Prunes, cooked, unsweetened, 1 cup	255	2	1	67
Prune juice, canned or bottled, 1 cup	195	1	Trace	49
Raisins, seedless				
1 cup, not pressed down	420	4	Trace	112
Packet, $\frac{1}{2}$ oz	40	Trace	Trace	11
Raspberries				
Raw, whole, 1 cup	70	1	1	17
Frozen, sweetened, 10-oz container	280	2	1	70
Rhubarb, cooked, added sugar, 1 cup	380	1	Trace	97
Strawberries				
Raw, whole berries, 1 cup	55	1	1	13
Frozen, sweetened, 1 container	310	1	1	79
Tangerine, 1 tangerine	40	1	Trace	10
Watermelon, 4" by 8" wedge with rind and seeds	110	2	1	27
GRAIN PRODUCTS				
Bagel, 3" diam., 1 bagel	165	6	2	28
Barley, pearled, light, uncooked, 1 cup	700	16	2	158
Bread				
Boston brown bread, canned, slice, $3\frac{1}{4}$" by $\frac{1}{2}$", 1 slice	95	2	1	21

Portion	Calories	Protein Grams	Fat	Carbo-hydrates Grams
Bread (Cont'd)				
Cracked-wheat bread ($\frac{3}{4}$ enriched wheat flour, $\frac{1}{4}$ cracked wheat)				
1 loaf	1,195	39	10	236
1 slice	65	2	1	13
Italian bread, enriched, 1 slice	85	3	Trace	17
Raisin bread, enriched, 1 slice	65	2	1	13
Rye bread, 1 slice	60	2	Trace	13
Pumpernickel, 1 slice	80	3	Trace	17
White bread, enriched				
Soft-crumb type, 1 slice	70	2	1	13
Firm-crumb type, 1 slice	65	2	1	12
Whole-wheat bread				
Soft-crumb type, 1 slice	65	3	1	14
Firm-crumb type, 1 slice	60	3	1	12
Breadcrumbs (enriched), dry, grated, 1 cup	390	13	5	73
Breakfast cereals				
Hot type, cooked				
Corn (hominy) grits, 1 cup	125	3	Trace	27
Oatmeal or rolled oats, 1 cup	130	5	2	23
Wheat, rolled, 1 cup	180	5	1	41
Wheat, whole-meal, 1 cup	110	4	1	23
Ready-to-eat				
Bran flakes (40% bran), 1 cup	105	4	1	28
Bran flakes with raisins, 1 cup	145	4	1	40
Corn flakes				
Regular, 1 cup	95	2	Trace	21
Sugar-coated, 1 cup	155	2	Trace	37
Corn, puffed, 1 cup	80	2	1	16
Oats, puffed, 1 cup	100	3	1	19
Rice, puffed				
Plain, 1 cup	60	1	Trace	13
Presweetened, 1 cup	115	1	0	26
Wheat flakes, 1 cup	105	3	Trace	24
Wheat, puffed				
Regular, 1 cup	55	2	Trace	12
Presweetened, 1 cup	140	3	Trace	33
Wheat, shredded, plain, 1 oblong biscuit or $\frac{1}{2}$ cup spoon-sized biscuits	90	2	1	20
Wheat germ, 1 tbsp	25	2	1	3
Buckwheat flour, light, sifted, 1 cup	340	6	1	78
Bulgur, canned, seasoned, 1 cup	245	8	4	44
Cakes made from mixes				
Coffeecake (7 $\frac{3}{4}$ " by 5 $\frac{5}{8}$ " by 1 $\frac{1}{4}$ "), $\frac{1}{6}$ of cake, 1 piece	230	5	7	38
Cupcakes, made with egg, milk, 2 $\frac{1}{2}$ " diam.				
Without icing, 1 cupcake	90	1	3	14
With chocolate icing, 1 cupcake	130	2	5	21
Devil's food with chocolate icing				
Whole, 2 layer cake (8" or 9" diam.), 1 cake	3,755	49	136	645
Piece, $\frac{1}{16}$ of cake	235	3	8	40
Cupcake, 2 $\frac{1}{2}$ " diam.	120	2	4	20
Gingerbread				
Whole cake (8" square)	1,575	18	39	291
Piece, $\frac{1}{9}$ of cake	175	2	4	32

Portion	Calories	Protein Grams	Fat	Carbo-hydrates Grams
Cakes made from mixes (Cont'd)				
White, 2 layer with chocolate icing				
Whole cake (8" or 9" diam.)	4,000	44	122	716
Piece, $\frac{1}{16}$ of cake	250	3	8	45
Yellow, 2 layer with chocolate icing				
Whole cake (8" or 9" diam.)	3,735	45	125	638
Piece, $\frac{1}{16}$ of cake	235	3	8	40
Cakes made from home recipes using enriched flour				
Boston cream pie with custard filling				
Whole cake (8" diam.)	2,490	41	78	412
Piece, $\frac{1}{12}$ of cake	210	3	6	34
Fruitcake, dark				
Loaf, 1 lb ($7\frac{1}{2}$" by 2" by $1\frac{1}{2}$")	1,720	22	69	271
Slice, $\frac{1}{30}$ of loaf	55	1	2	9
Plain, sheet cake				
Without icing				
Whole cake (9" square)	2,830	35	108	434
Piece, $\frac{1}{9}$ of cake	315	4	12	48
With uncooked white icing				
Whole cake (9" square)	4,020	37	129	694
Piece, $\frac{1}{9}$ of cake	445	4	14	77
Pound				
Loaf, $8\frac{1}{2}$" by $3\frac{1}{2}$" by $3\frac{1}{4}$"	2,725	31	170	273
Slice, $\frac{1}{17}$ of loaf	160	2	10	16
Spongecake				
Whole cake ($9\frac{3}{4}$" diam. tube cake)	2,345	60	45	427
Piece, $\frac{1}{12}$ of cake	195	5	4	36
Cookies made with enriched flour				
Brownies with nuts				
Home-prepared, $1\frac{3}{4}$" by $1\frac{3}{4}$" by $\frac{7}{8}$" piece				
From home recipe	95	1	6	10
From commercial recipe	85	1	4	13
Frozen, with chocolate icing, $1\frac{1}{2}$" by $1\frac{3}{4}$" by $\frac{7}{8}$" piece	105	1	5	15
Chocolate chip				
Commercial, $2\frac{1}{4}$" diam., $\frac{3}{8}$" thick, 4 cookies	200	2	9	29
From home recipe, $2\frac{1}{3}$" diam., 4 cookies	205	2	12	24
Fig bars, square ($1\frac{5}{8}$" by $1\frac{5}{8}$" by $\frac{3}{8}$") or rectangular ($1\frac{1}{2}$" by $1\frac{3}{4}$" by $\frac{1}{2}$"), 4 cookies	200	2	3	42
Gingersnaps, 2" diam, $\frac{1}{4}$" thick, 4 cookies	90	2	2	22
Macaroons, $2\frac{3}{4}$" diam., $\frac{1}{4}$" thick, 2 cookies	180	2	9	25
Oatmeal with raisins, $2\frac{5}{8}$" diam., $\frac{1}{4}$" thick, 4 cookies	235	3	8	38
Plain, prepared from commercial chilled dough, $2\frac{1}{2}$" diam., $\frac{1}{4}$" thick, 4 cookies	240	2	12	31
Sandwich type (chocolate or vanilla), $1\frac{3}{4}$" diam., $\frac{3}{8}$" thick, 4 cookies	200	2	9	28
Vanilla wafers, $1\frac{3}{4}$" diam., $\frac{1}{4}$" thick, 10 cookies	185	2	6	30
Cornmeal, cooked, 1 cup	120	3	Trace	26
Crackers				
Graham, 2 crackers	55	1	1	10
Rye wafers, 2 wafers	45	2	Trace	10
Saltines, 4 crackers or 1 packet	50	1	1	8

Portion	Calories	Protein Grams	Fat	Carbo-hydrates Grams
Danish pastry without fruit or nuts, piece about 4¼" diam. by 1" thick, 1 pastry	275	5	15	30
Macaroni, enriched, cooked (cut lengths, elbows, shells)				
Firm stage (hot), 1 cup	190	7	1	39
Tender stage				
Cold macaroni, 1 cup	115	4	Trace	24
Hot macaroni, 1 cup	155	5	1	32
Macaroni (enriched) and cheese, canned, 1 cup	230	9	10	26
Muffins made with enriched flour				
Blueberry, 2⅜" diam., 1½" high, 1 muffin	110	3	4	17
Bran, 1 muffin	105	3	4	17
Corn, 2⅜" diam., 1½" high, 1 muffin	125	3	4	19
Noodles (egg), cooked, 1 cup	200	7	2	37
Pancakes (4" diam.)				
Buckwheat, made from mix, 1 cake	55	2	2	6
Plain, made from mix, 1 cake	60	2	2	9
Pies				
Apple, 1 section	345	3	15	51
Blueberry, 1 section	325	3	15	47
Cherry, 1 section	350	4	15	52
Custard, 1 section	285	8	14	30
Lemon Meringue, 1 section	305	4	12	45
Peach, 1 section	345	3	14	52
Pumpkin, 1 section	275	5	15	32
Pizza (cheese) baked, 4¾" section, 1 section	145	6	4	22
Popcorn, popped, with oil and salt, 1 cup	40	1	2	5
Pretzels				
Dutch, 1 pretzel	60	2	1	12
Thin, twisted, 10 pretzels	235	6	3	46
Stick, 10 pretzels	10	Trace	Trace	2
Rice				
Instant, ready-to-serve, 1 cup	180	4	Trace	40
Long grain, cooked, 1 cup	225	4	Trace	50
Rolls				
Brown-and-serve, 1 roll	85	2	2	14
Cloverleaf, 1 roll	85	2	2	15
Frankfurter and hamburger, 1 roll	120	3	2	21
Hard, 1 roll	155	5	2	30
Spaghetti, cooked				
Firm stage, "al dente," 1 cup	190	7	1	39
Tender stage, 1 cup	155	5	1	32
Spaghetti in tomato sauce with cheese				
Home recipe, 1 cup	260	9	9	37
Canned, 1 cup	190	6	2	39
Spaghetti with meat balls and tomato sauce				
Home recipe, 1 cup	330	19	12	39
Canned, 1 cup	260	12	10	29
Waffles, 7" diam., from mix, 1 waffle	205	7	8	27
Wheat flour				
All-purpose or family, sifted, 1 cup	420	12	1	88
Cake or pastry, sifted, 1 cup	350	7	1	76
Self-rising, unsifted, 1 cup	440	12	1	93
Whole-wheat, 1 cup	400	16	2	85

Portion	Calories	Protein Grams	Fat	Carbo-hydrates Grams
LEGUMES (DRY), NUTS, SEEDS: RELATED PRODUCTS				
Almonds, shelled				
Chopped (about 130 almonds), 1 cup	775	24	70	25
Slivered, not pressed down, (about 115 almonds), 1 cup	690	21	62	22
Beans, dry				
Common varieties as Great Northern, navy, lentils, and others: cooked, drained, 1 cup	210	14	1	38
Limas, cooked, 1 cup	260	16	1	49
Blackeye peas, dry, cooked, 1 cup	190	13	1	35
Brazil nuts, shelled (6–8 large kernels, 1 oz)	185	4	19	3
Cashew nuts, roasted in oil, 1 oz	785	24	64	41
Coconut meat, shredded or grated, 1 cup	275	3	28	8
Peanuts, roasted in oil, salted, 1 cup	840	37	72	27
Peanut butter, 1 tbsp	95	4	8	3
Peas, split, dry, cooked, 1 cup	230	16	1	42
Pecans, chopped or pieces (about 120 large halves), 1 cup	810	11	84	17
Pumpkin and squash kernels, dry, hulled, 1 cup	775	41	65	21
Sunflower seeds, dry, hulled, 1 cup	810	35	69	29
Walnuts, English, chopped, 1 cup	780	18	77	19
SUGARS				
Sugar				
Brown, pressed down, 1 cup	820	0	0	212
White, granulated, 1 tbsp	45	0	0	12
VEGETABLE AND VEGETABLE PRODUCTS				
Asparagus, cooked, cut up				
From raw, 1 cup	30	3	Trace	5
From frozen, 1 cup	40	6	Trace	6
Spears				
From raw, 4 spears	10	1	Trace	2
From frozen, 4 spears	15	2	Trace	2
Beans				
Lima, frozen, cooked				
Thick-seeded types (ford-hooks), 1 cup	170	10	Trace	32
Thin-seeded types (baby limas), 1 cup	210	13	Trace	40
Kidney beans, canned red, 1 cup	230	15	1	42
Snap				
Green or yellow (or wax), cooked				
From raw, 1 cup	30	2	Trace	7
From frozen, 1 cup	35	2	Trace	8
Bean sprouts (mung), raw or cooked, 1 cup	35	4	Trace	7
Beets				
Cooked, drained, peeled				
Whole, 2" diam., 2 beets	30	1	Trace	7
Diced or sliced, 1 cup	55	2	Trace	12
Canned				
Whole, 1 cup	60	2	Trace	14
Diced or sliced, 1 cup	65	2	Trace	15

Portion	Calories	Protein Grams	Fat	Carbo-hydrates Grams
Beet greens, leaves and stems, cooked, drained, 1 cup	25	2	Trace	5
Blackeye peas, cooked				
From raw, 1 cup	180	13	1	30
From frozen, 1 cup	220	15	1	40
Broccoli, cooked				
From raw				
Stalk, medium size, 1 stalk	45	6	1	8
Stalks cut into $\frac{1}{2}$" pieces, 1 cup	40	5	Trace	7
From frozen				
Stalk, $4\frac{1}{2}$" to 5" long, 1 stalk	10	1	Trace	1
Chopped, 1 cup	50	5	Trace	9
Brussels sprouts, cooked				
From raw, 1 cup	55	7	1	10
From frozen, 1 cup	50	5	Trace	10
Cabbage				
Raw, shredded or sliced, 1 cup	15	1	Trace	4
Cooked, drained, 1 cup	30	2	Trace	6
Cabbage, celery (also called Chinese), raw, 1 cup	10	1	Trace	2
Cabbage, white mustard (also called bokchoy or pakchoy), cooked, drained, 1 cup	25	2	Trace	4
Carrots				
Raw, 1 carrot	30	1	Trace	7
Cooked (crosswise cuts), 1 cup	50	1	Trace	11
Cauliflower, cooked, 1 cup	30	3	Trace	5
Celery, 1 stalk	5	Trace	Trace	2
Collards, cooked				
From raw, 1 cup	65	7	1	10
From frozen, 1 cup	50	5	1	10
Corn				
Cooked				
From raw, 1 ear	70	2	1	16
From frozen:				
Ear, 5" long, 1 ear	120	4	1	27
Kernels, 1 cup	130	5	1	31
Canned				
Cream style, 1 cup	210	5	2	51
Whole kernel				
Vacuum pack, 1 cup	175	5	1	43
Wet pack, 1 cup	140	4	1	33
Dandelion greens, cooked, 1 cup	35	2	1	7
Endive, curly (including escarole), raw, small pieces, 1 cup	10	1	Trace	2
Kale, cooked, 1 cup	45	5	1	7
Lettuce, raw:				
Butterhead, Boston types				
Head, 5" diam., 1 head	25	2	Trace	4
Crisphead, Iceberg type				
Head, 6" diam., 1 head	70	5	1	16
Wedge, $\frac{1}{4}$ of head, 1 wedge	20	1	Trace	4
Looseleaf (bunching varieties including romaine or cos), chopped or shredded pieces, 1 cup	10	1	Trace	2

Portion	Calories	Protein Grams	Fat	Carbo- hydrates Grams
Mushrooms, raw, sliced or chopped, 1 cup	20	2	Trace	3
Mustard greens, cooked, 1 cup	30	3	1	6
Okra pods, cooked, 10 pods	30	2	Trace	6
Onions				
Raw, chopped, 1 cup	65	3	Trace	15
Cooked, 1 cup	60	3	Trace	14
Parsnips, cooked, 1 cup	100	2	1	23
Peas, green				
Canned, 1 cup	150	8	1	29
Frozen, cooked, 1 cup	110	8	Trace	19
Potatoes, cooked:				
Baked, 1 potato	145	4	Trace	33
Boiled, 1 potato	90	3	Trace	20
French-fried				
Prepared from raw, 10 strips	135	2	7	18
Frozen, oven heated, 10 strips	110	2	4	17
Hash brown, prepared from frozen, 1 cup	345	3	18	45
Mashed, prepared from raw				
Milk added, 1 cup	135	4	2	27
Milk and butter added, 1 cup	195	4	9	26
Dehydrated flakes, water, milk, butter added, 1 cup	195	4	7	30
Potato salad, made with cooked salad dressing, 1 cup	250	7	7	41
Pumpkin, canned, 1 cup	80	2	1	19
Sauerkraut, canned, 1 cup	40	2	Trace	9
Spinach, cooked				
From raw, 1 cup	40	5	1	6
From frozen, 1 cup	45	6	1	8
Squash, cooked				
Summer (all varieties), 1 cup	30	2	Trace	7
Winter (all varieties), 1 cup	130	4	1	32
Sweet potatoes				
Baked in skin, peeled, 1 potato	160	2	1	37
Boiled in skin, peeled, 1 potato	170	3	1	40
Canned, solid pack (mashed), 1 cup	275	5	1	63
Tomatoes:				
Raw, 1 tomato	25	1	Trace	6
Canned, solids and liquid, 1 cup	50	2	Trace	10
Tomato juice, canned, 1 cup	45	2	Trace	10
Turnips, cooked, diced, 1 cup	35	1	Trace	8
Turnip greens, cooked				
From raw, 1 cup	30	3	Trace	5
From frozen (chopped), 1 cup	40	4	Trace	6
Vegetables, mixed, frozen, cooked, 1 cup	115	6	1	24

Index

Abraham, Sydney, 235
Acetoacetic acid, 47
Acid foods, starches should not be combined with, 65
Acid-forming foods, 13
Acorn squash, 89
Addicting foods, 48
Aerobics, 142–44
Aging process, 19
  carbohydrates and, 35
  exercises and, 142
  stress and, 171
  protein intake and, 24, 25
  turning back, 20–21
Air pollution, 164
Alcoholic beverages, 75–77, 83
Allen, James, 231
American Natural Hygiene Society, 16–17, 80–81
Amino acids, 23, 30–31
Amphetamines, 36, 174
Anabolism, 46, 172
Anaerobics, 142
Appearance, new eating plan and, 60
  See also Younger appearance
Appetite, 69–71
Apples, mozzarella cheese and, 114
Apricot Fluff, 111
Asparagus, 87
Aspirin, 170
Atherosclerosis, 75
Athletes, natural carbohydrates and, 31–32
Avocado, 65
  dressing, 99
  Pitacado, 117
  prime, 89

Banana (s) :
  –Coconut Cream Pie, 117
  Milk Shake, 112
  prime, 89
  storage of, 92
Bandy, Way, 69
Barbiturates, 173–74
Bathing, 186
  in Born-Again Body Program, 197, 205
  fasting and, 51
Bean (s) , 65, 87
  Soup, Black, 103
Bellows of Life exercise, 158
Beverages, 62, 72–79
  for entertaining, 114
  recipes for, 111–13
  See also Specific beverages
Bibb lettuce, 88
Black Bean Soup, 103
Blake, William, 207
Blood cells, red, alcohol and, 76–77
Blood pressure:
  high, 62, 74
  sunlight and, 167
Bloom, Walter, 236
Body odors, 219
Born-Again Body Program, 5, 7, 193–231
  approach to living changed by, 15
  fasting in, 5, 14, 193–201
  journal kept while on, 194, 196–98, 200, 215, 219, 220, 222, 226, 229
  "low" at start of, 194
  preview of, 14–15
  See also Natural Carbohydrate Diet; and specific subjects
Born-Again Salad, basic, 96

Boston lettuce, 88
Brain, 33
    alcohol and, 76
    fasting and, 47
Breakfast:
    menus for. *See* Menus
    skipping, 119, 175
Breath, bad, 164
Breathing, 5, 159–66, 214
    aerobics and, 142
    exercise and, 165
    improving your, 165–66
    overweight and, 165
    polluted air, 164
    shallow, 160
    smoking and, 164–66
    stale air, 164
Breathing exercises:
    Bellows of Life, 158
    complete breath, 161–62
    deep breath, 161
    for insomnia, 175
Broccoli, 87
    Casserole, 104–5
    for finger salad, 97
    storage of, 91
Brussels sprouts, 87–88
Buckwheat groats, 94
Buttercrunch Salad, 98
Butternut squash, 89

Caffeine, 73
Cake, Uncooked Fruit, 81
Calisthenics, 142
Calories:
    "empty," 33
    exercise and, 141
    in Protein Counter, 26
    weight loss and, 42–43
Camps, summer, 81
Cancer, 74
    vegetarianism and, 237–38
Cantaloupe, 90
Carbohydrates (natural carbohydrates) ,
        5, 10, 12–14, 20
    aging process and, 35
    in American diet, 32, 33
    athletes and, 31–32
    central nervous system and, 34–35
    as energy source, 23–24, 31–33
    fast-energy, 239
    as fiber source, 34
    heart and, 34
    junk food and, 33
    metabolism of, 20
    as protein source, 33–34
    as protein-sparing, 33

Carbohydrates (*Continued*)
    "sweet tooth" and, 35
    vitamins and minerals provided by,
        34
    water content of, 34
    weight gain and, 34
Carbon dioxide, 160, 163, 168
Cardiomyopathy, 76
Carlyle, Thomas, 219
Carrell, Alexis, 46
Carrot (s) , 88
    juice, 112
Casserole (s) :
    Cheese, 114–15
    recipes for, 108–9
Catabolism, 172
Cauliflower, 87
    cheese-topped, 106
Cause and effect, law of, 219
Celery, 100
Cells:
    breathing and, 163
    fasting and, 46
Central nervous system, carbohydrates
        and, 34–35
Cereals. *See* Grains and grain products
Change, 3–5
Cheese, 238, 239
    Casserole, 114–15
    for entertaining, 114
    finger salads with, 100
    -topped Cauliflower, 106
    See also Specific cheeses
Chemicals (chemical additives) , 21, 62
Child, C. M., 46
Children, 9
    maturation rate of, 19
    New Lifetime Eating Plan and, 80–82
    protein and, 23
    vacations away from, 176
Chocolate, 73, 74
Choice, of happy way of life, 178
Cigarette smoking, 164–66
Circulation:
    exercise and, 143
    respiration and, 159–60
Coal-tar derivatives, 73
Coffee, 174
    fasting and, 52
    harmfulness of, 73–74
    substitute, 119
Cola drinks, 174
Complete breath, 161–62
Connor, William E., 36
Contentment, 178
Cooking, 60, 92–94
    water in, 93
Cookware, 92–93

Corn, 88
  fresh sweet Kentucky style, 109
  soup, creamy, 102
Cottage Cheese:
  dressing, 99
  and Sour Cream Dip
Crackers, Cheese Tray with, 114
Cream Pie, Banana-Coconut, 117
Cucumber (s) , 88
  masque, 226
Cynopep, 119

Dairy products, protein grams in, 27
  (chart)
DeWaard, Fritz, 19
Deamination, 24, 172
Deep breath, 161
Depression, 169
Desserts, recipes for, 116–17
Detoxification, 5
Dey, Frederick van Rensselaer, 225
Diaphragm, 159–61
Diet (s) :
  fad, 235–36
  fertility problems and, 188–89
  "go on a," as false idea, 4
  Joy Gross's personal, 33
  protein-sparing, 37, 236
  puberty and, 19
  sex and, 188
  vegetarian. *See* Vegetarian diet
  See also Natural Carbohydrate Diet
Digestion:
  food combining and, 63–64
  of milk, 75
  See also Food combining
Dinner, menus for. *See* Menus
Dip, Sour Cream and Cottage Cheese,
  113
Diuretic (s) , 36–37, 170
  coffee as, 74
Di Vries, Arnold, 50
Dizziness, fasting and, 50
Dressings, salad, 95, 98–100
Drinking. *See* Beverages
Drugs, 21
  sunlight and, 170
Dyer, Wayne, 203, 221

Eating habits, 5
  hungry, eating when, 20–21
  night-, 175
  See also Lifetime Eating Plan
Eating Plan, *see* Lifetime Eating Plan
Eggplant:
  Baked Stuffed, 104
  Steak, 105
  Stuffed, 105–6

Eggs, 238
  as meat substitute, 120–21
  protein grams in, 27 (chart)
Emerson, Ralph Waldo, 215, 224
Enemas, fasting and, 51
Energy:
  breathing and, 163–64
  natural carbohydrates as best source
    of, 23–24, 31–33
  sex and, 186
  sun as source of, 167–70
Entertaining, recipes and suggestions for,
  113–115
Exercise (s) , 14, 15, 18, 21
  aging and, 142
  breathing and, 165. *See also* Breathing
    exercises
  drinking water after, 78
  fasting and, 51
  happiness and, 181–82
  heart and, 141–43, 165
  sex and, 186
  sexual, 223–24
  slow hand meditation, 221
  stomach-control, 224–25
  stomach flattener, 221–22
  for stress, 158
  stretching and bending, 195
  types of, 142–43
  Yvonne's Head-to-Toe Shape-up, 147–
    58

Face, cucumber masque for, 226
Facial, yogurt, 213–14
Facial exercise, 217
Fad diets, 235–36
Fast-food industry, 235
Fasting, 5, 61
  advantages of, 236
  Born-Again Body Program and, 5, 14,
    193–201, 215
  drinking water during, 50
  fertility problems and, 188–89
  historical background of, 45–46
  at home, 48–55
  for insomniacs, 174
  Joy Gross's experience with, 10, 11
  Joy Gross's mother's experience with,
    8–9
  looking younger and, 14
  metabolism and, 47–48
  one day every week, 175
  personal experiences with, 17, 38–41
  protein-sparing, 37
  psyching yourself up to begin, 49–50
  re-feeding plan after, 53–55, 199, 201–2
  rejuvenation and, 46
  retreats, 240

Fasting (*Continued*)
  sex response and, 187–88
  shampooing while, 198
  starving differentiated from, 48
  symptoms that may occur during, 50–51
  three-day, 52–53
Fat (body), 141
  fasting and, 47–48
  See also Overweight
Fat (s), 32
  protein grams in, 28 (chart)
  protein intake and, 24
  saturated, 20
Feldman, Sol, 38–39
Fertility problems, fasting and, 188–89
Fiber, carbohydrates as source of, 34
Figs, fresh, 90
Finger Salad, 97, 100
Fish, 119
  as meat substitute, 119–21
  protein grams in, 27 (chart)
  protein intake and daily eating of, 29
Five-Fruit Sundae, 116
Flour, refined white, 33
Food (s):
  addicting, 48
  combining, 62–69
  combining, chart, 63
  combining, menus, 67–68
  live versus dead, 20
  minimum, as adequate, 20
  neutral, 67
  Plan. *See* Lifetime Eating Plan
  sex and, 186–87
  whole, 61
  See also Menus
Food and Nutrition Board, 25–26
Friends' homes, eating at, 83
  See also Parties
Fructose (fruit sugar), 32, 35
  food combining and, 66
Fruit (s)
  Ambrosia, Fresh, 117
  cake, uncooked, 81–82
  dried, 92
  juices, 77–78, 111–12
  mail-order sources for, 241
  mono-meals of, 68–69
  prime, 86–87, 89–91
  protein grams in, 29 (chart)
  recipes for, 110–11
  Special, Fresh, 110
  storage of, 92
  sugar. *See* Fructose

Gandhi, Mahatma, 61–62
Glasser, Ronald, 73

Glucose, 33, 163
  fasting and, 47, 52
Goals, 181, 182
Goldstein, Jack, 41–42
Graham, Sylvester, 45
Grains and grain products, 33
  cooking, 94
  protein grams in, 28 (chart)
  recipes for, 107–9
  whole, 33, 34
Grapefruit, 89–90
Grapes, 90
Gratification, 178
Gray, Dina, 189–90
Gray, Martin, 189–90, 216
Green Bean Paté, 103–4
Green Goddess Drink, 112
Green Pea Soup, 102
Green peppers, 88
Grooming tips, natural, 15, 195–96
Gross, Harry, 16–17
Gross, Joy, 7–11
Gross, Robert, 4, 16–17
Gross, Sara, 17

Habits, life-denying, 4
Hair, dry, 222
Happiness, 177–82
  choosing, 178
  components of, 178–79
  health and, 178
  learning the secret of your own, 21
  longevity and, 177–78
  physical self and, 179–81
  rules for starting on road to, 180–82
Harris, Sidney J., 226
Hazzard, Linda Burfield, 45
Headaches, 79
  alcohol and, 77
  coffee and, 74
  fasting and, 50
Health:
  happiness and, 178
  as resulting from a total way of life, 11
  vegetarianism and, 237
Heart:
  alcohol and, 76
  carbohydrates and, 34
  coffee and, 74
  exercise and, 141–43, 165
  fasting and, 50
Heart disease, 34
  milk and, 75
  vegetarianism and, 237
Herb tea, 119
Herbal steam, 205
High blood pressure, 62, 74
Hill, Napoleon, 181

Hilton, Sam, 179–80
Hors d'oeuvres, 113
Hubbard squash, 89
Hull, Raymond, 217
Hunger (hungry) , 69–70
    eating only when, 20–21
Hygienists, natural, 9, 10, 17

Ice Cream, Tropical Suprise, 116
Insomniacs, 174–75
Isometrics, 142
Isotonics, 142, 143

Jagger, Bianca, 208
Jogging, 18, 142–46, 174
Johnson, Jack, 38
Jordan, William George, 178
Juices, fruit, 32
Jump rope, 143
Junk food, as "empty calories," 33

Kasha, 94
    Casserole, 108–9
Ketones, 48
Ketosis, 48
Kidneys, 37
Kiev peasants, longevity of, 177
Krishnamurti, J., 200, 230
Kübler-Ross, Elisabeth, 204
Kutter Cheese Company, 100

Lasagna, Whole-wheat, 115
Legumes, protein grams in, 27 (chart)
Lentil stew, 106
Lettuce, 88
Lifespan:
    normal, 19
    See also Longevity
Lifetime cookware, 93
Lifetime Eating Plan, 15, 45, 59–61, 194
    advantages of, 60
    appetite and, 69–71
    children and, 80–81
    helping your mate to switch over to, 82
    See also Born-Again Body Program;
        Food, combining
Linguine, Delicious Whole-wheat, 109
Liver (organ) , 37
    alcohol and, 77
Longevity, 4–5
    balanced and whole approach needed
        for, 16–17
    happiness and, 177–78
    as resulting from a total way of life, 11
    turning back your time clock, 20–21

Longevity *(Continued)*
    of Ukrainian peasants, 177
    See also Lifespan
Looking younger, 20
Loufa, 209
Lunch:
    menus for. *See* Menus
    recipes for, 117–18
Lungs, 160
    smoking and, 164
    See also Breathing

Magical Liquid exercise, 158
Mandala, 199–200
Mango (es) , 90
    Divine, 110–11
Mann, George, 141
Mansfield, Joan, 41
Masai tribe, 141
Massage, in Born-Again Body Program,
    200–1
Matson, Floyd W., 228
Maturation rate, 19
Mayer, Jean, 20, 23, 31, 34
McKay, Clive, 48–49
Meat:
    abstaining from, 119
    cancer and, 237–38
    food combining and, 65–66
    protein grams in, 27 (chart)
    protein intake and daily eating of, 29
    sun-energy and, 168
Meditation, 175, 205
    slow hand, 221
Melanocytes, 167
Melons, 90
Menstrual period:
    first, 19, 20
    irregularities of, 189
Mental rest, 172–73
Menus, 119–36
    first week, 122–125
    second week, 125–28
    third week, 129–32
    fourth week, 132–36
Metabolism, 11, 37, 172
    alcohol and, 76
    carbohydrate, 20
    fasting, 37, 47–48
    of protein, 12, 20
    vegetarianism and, 238
Methionine, 31
Milk, 74–75, 238–39
    Shake, Banana, 112
Miller, Lowell G., 160–61
Millet, 109
Mindset, 15
Minerals, 34, 79

Mono-meal plan, 68–69
Montaigne, 19
Morris, Fay, 17–18
Mozzarella Cheese, Apples and, 114
Muscles, 33
Mushrooms, Stuffed, 113–14

Natural Carbohydrate Diet, 12, 14, 22–35
Natural carbohydrates:
    nutritionists current views on, 22–23
    as percentage of your diet, 22
Natural Hygienists, 9, 10, 17
Nature, 5
Nausea, fasting and, 50
Nearing, Scott, 223
Nectarines, 91
Negative living patterns, 4, 14
New Lifetime Eating Plan. See Lifetime
    Eating Plan
Nibble Packs, 137
Night Thoughts, 15
    See also Born-Again Body Program
Nitrogen, 24, 30–31
Nut butters, recipe for, 111
Nutrition, breathing and, 159
Nutrition and Human Needs, U.S. Sen-
    ate Committee on, 32, 34
Nuts, 119
    mail-order sources for
    protein grams in, 27–28 (chart)
    storage of, 92

Odors, body, 219
Oils:
    protein grams in, 28 (chart)
    for salad dressings, 95
Onions, 88
Oranges, 78, 89–90
Overweight (obesity), 36–43, 235
    appetite and, 70
    artificial ways of dealing with, 36–37
    breathing and, 165
    fasting to overcome, 37–42
    menus for, 119
    sex and, 186–87
    See also Weight gain; Weight loss
Oxygen, 159, 160
    See also Breathing

Papayas, 90
Parsley, 88
    storage of, 91–92
Parsnips, 88
Parties:
    natural foods at, 81–84
    recipes for, 113–15

Patterfield, Susan, 40–41
Pawling Health Manor, 4, 5, 49, 187
Peaches, 91
Pears, 91
Peas, 65, 87
Pep talks to oneself, 175
Perkins, Charles Eliot, 74
Pero, 119
Photosynthesis, 168
Physical rest, 172–75
Physiological rest, 173, 175–76
Pineapple (s) , 91
    Cooler, 112–13
    Delight, 110
Pitacado, 117
Pituitary gland, 167
Plants, sunlight and, 167, 169
Pleasure, 178–79, 184–85
    See also Sex
Plums, 91
Positive Thinking, 14
Posture, 196
Potatoes, 88
Preservatives, 78
Problems, handling, 175
Protein:
    "complete," 30
    food combining and, 64–66
    metabolism of, 12, 20
    myths about, 23–24, 30
    natural carbohydrates as source of, 33–
        34
    non-meat sources of, 239
    recommended dietary allowance for, 26
    –sparing diet (or fast) , 37, 236
Protein Counter, 12, 26
    sample chart, 27–29
Protein Intake, 6, 10, 12
    aging effect of excessive, 24, 25
    of children, 23
    finding out your, 24–25
    meat and fish in daily diet and, 29
    nutritionists recommending lower, 22–
        23
    overdosing on, 20
    vegetarianism and, 238
    weight gain and, 24
    See also Protein Counter
Proxmire, William, 18–19
Psoriasis, 8, 9, 10, 169
Puberty, diet and, 19
Puretz, Donald, 144–45
Pyridine, 74–75

Rainbow salad, 97
Re-feeding plan after fasting, 53–55
Reich, Charles, 198

Rejuvenation, fasting and, 46
Respiration. *See* Breathing
Rest, 21, 171–76
    fasting and, 50
    sex and, 186
Restaurants, 82–83, 199, 206–7
Rica-dog, 117
Rice (brown) , recipes for, 107–8
Ringer, Robert J., 206, 209
Romaine lettuce, 88
Running, 142–46
Rush, David, 237

Sagan, Carl, 224
Salad (s) , 95–98
    dressings for, 95, 98–100
    in restaurants, 82–83
Salt, 62
    in salads, 96
Salter, Andrew, 164
Salty foods, 72–73
Satisfaction, 178
Saturated fats, 20
Sauce, for Whole-wheat Lasagne, 115
Saunas, fasting and, 51
Scavullo, Francesco, 227
Schaffenberg, John A., 238
Scrimshaw, Nevin, 47
Seeds, 119
    storage of, 92
Self-discipline, 208, 222, 223
Self-improvement, 181, 182
Selye, Hans, 19, 171
Sensory rest, 173, 175
Sex (sexual pleasure) , 183–90
    alcohol and, 77
    diet and, 188
    fasting and, 187–88
    food and, 186–87
    rightness of, 185–86
Shampooing, 227
    dry hair, 222
    hair, 198
Shelton, Herbert, 19, 20, 44, 50, 64, 188–89, 222, 224
Sherman's Arcadia Soup Base, 96
Shore, Dinah, 213
Showering, 197
Sinclair, Upton, 46
Skin, 69, 228
    sunlight and, 169–70
Sleep:
    drug-induced, 173–74
    fasting and, 52
    See also Insomniacs; Rest
Smith, Bill, 39
Smith, Nathan, 20, 34

Smoking, 164–66
    fasting and, 51
    quitting, 21
Snacks, 122–36
    Nibble Packs with, 137
Soap, 215
Soft drinks, 32, 73
Soup (s) , 101–3
    base for, 96
Sour Cream and Cottage Cheese Dip, 113
Soviet Union, 177
Spaghetti. *See* Linguine
Spanish casserole, 108
Spinach, 88
    salad, 97
Squash:
    à la Joy, 105
    summer, 88–89
    winter, 89
Starches, 32
    food combining and, 65–67
    proteins should not be combined with, 65
Steam baths, fasting and, 51
Steaming vegetables, 93–94
Stew, lentil, 106
Stimulants, 174
Stomach:
    –control exercise, 224
    –flattener exercise, 221–22
Stress:
    aging process and, 19
    exercises to combat, 158
    maturation and, 20
    rest and, 171
Stretching exercises, 195
Struggle, 210
Stuffed Mushrooms, 113–14
Sucrose (refined sugar) , 33, 73
    per capita consumption of, 32
Sugar (s) :
    food combining and, 66–67
    fruit, 32
    per capita consumption of, 32
    refined. *See* Sucrose
    Summer camp, 81
    See also Glucose
Sun (sunlight) , 13, 167–70
Sunbathing, 169–70
    fasting and, 51
Sunburst salad, 98
Sundae, Five-Fruit, 116
Sweet potatoes, 89

Tangerines, 90
Tannic acid, 74
Tea, 73, 74, 174
    herb, 119

Teenagers, protein needs of, 25
Theobromine, 73, 74
Thinking, alcohol impairs, 77
Theoreau, Henry David, 196, 213, 224
Theroux, Phyllis, 202
Tokay grapes, 90
Tomato (es) , 89
  dressing, 99
Toothpaste, 216
Toxins, drinking water and, 78–79
  fasting and, 46, 47
Trall, Russell J., 45
Tropical Surprise Ice Cream, 116
Tropical Treat, 112
Turnips, 88
Tutor, E. E., 146

Vacation (s) , 176
  retreats, 240
Vagina:
  cleansing, 210
  exercise for, 223–24
Vegebase, 96, 118
Vege-shaker, 118
Vegetable (s) :
  amino-acid balance in protein from,
    30–31
  in casseroles, 103–7
  mail-order sources for, 241
  prime, 86–89
  protein grams in, 28 (chart)
  as protein sources, 31
  salad, mixed, 96
  soup, 101–2
  steaming, 93–94
  storage of, 91–92
  sun-energy and, 168
Vegetarian diet (vegetarianism) , 18, 61–
  62
  arguments in favor of, 237–38
  excessive protein intake and, 29–30
Vinegar, 96

Vitamins, carbohydrates and, 34
Vitamin D, 169, 170
Vitamin pills, 13
Vomiting, fasting and, 50
Von Furstenberg, Diane, 214

Water:
  carbohydrates and, 34
  in cooking, 93
  fasting and, 50
  proportion of, in your system, 72
  salty foods and, 72–73
  spring, 50
Watercress:
  Special Salad, 98
  storage of, 91–92
Watermelon, 90
Weight gain:
  carbohydrates and, 34
  protein intake and, 24
  See also Overweight
Weight loss, by fasting, 37–42, 47, 237
Whole foods, 61
Wholeness, 178, 185
Whole-wheat Lasagna, 115
Whole-wheat Linguine, 109
Wild and Wonderful Rice, 107–8
Winter squash, 89

Yams, 89
Yogurt, 239
Yogurt facial, 213–14
Young, Vernon R., 47
Younger appearance, 20
Yvonne, 142–43, 146–47
Yvonne's Head-to-Toe Shape-up, 147–58

Zucchini, Stuffed, 105–6